Certified Coding Specialist– Physician-based (CCS–P) Exam Preparation

Third Edition

Anita C. Hazelwood, MLS, RHIA, FAHIMA

Lynn Kuehn, MS, RHIA, CCS-P, FAHIMA

Carol A. Venable, MPH, RHIA, FAHIMA

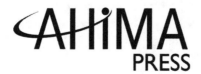

AHIMA
PRESS

ISBN 978-1-58426-265-7

AHIMA Product No. AC400210

AHIMA Staff:
Katherine Greenock, Editorial and Production Coordinator
Tanai S. Nelson, RHIT, CCS, CCS–P, Technical Review
Ashley Sullivan, Assistant Editor
Pamela Woolf, Developmental Editor
Ken Zielske, Director of Publications

All information contained within this book, including Web sites and regulatory information, was current and valid as of the date of publication. However, Web page addresses and the information on them may change or disappear at any time and for any number of reasons. The user is encouraged to perform his or her own general Web searches to locate any site addresses listed here that are no longer valid.

All products mentioned in this book are either trademarks of the companies referenced in this book, registered trademarks of the companies of the companies referenced in this book, or neither.

This book is sold, as is, without warranty of any kind, either express or implied. While every precaution has been taken in the preparation of this book, the publisher and author assume no responsibility for errors or omissions. Neither is any liability assumed for damages resulting from the use of the information or instructions contained herein. It is further stated that the publisher and author are not responsible for any damage or loss to your data or your equipment that results directly or indirectly from your use of this book.

AHIMA certifications are administered by the AHIMA Commission on Certification (COC). The COC does not contribute to, review or endorse any review books, review sessions, study guides or other exam preparatory activities. Use of this product for AHIMA certification exam preparation in no way guarantees an exam candidate will earn a passing score on the exam.

American Health Information Management Association
233 North Michigan Avenue, 21st Floor
Chicago, Illinois 60601-5809

ahima.org

Contents

ON THE CD-ROM
Practice Questions with Answers
Practice Exam 1 with Answers
Practice Exam 2 with Answers
Practice Exam 3 with Answers

About the Authors

Carol A. Venable, MPH, RHIA, FAHIMA, is a department head and a professor at the University of Louisiana at Lafayette, and **Anita C. Hazelwood, MLS, RHIA, FAHIMA,** is a professor at the same university. Their book, *ICD-10-CM Preview,* was first published by AHIMA in 2003 and was updated in 2004 with a new chapter on ICD-10-PCS.

Both authors have conducted numerous coding workshops at the local, state, and national levels. Moreover, they have published articles in *Educational Perspectives in Health Information Management,* in addition to serving on its editorial review board, and in the *Journal of AHIMA.*

Active volunteers of AHIMA, Ms. Venable and Ms. Hazelwood are members of the Assembly on Education and the Society for Clinical Coding and have served on the board of the Assembly on Education. Ms. Hazelwood also has served on the board of the Society for Clinical Coding.

Lynn Kuehn, MS, RHIA, CCS-P, FAHIMA, is president of Kuehn Consulting in Waukesha, Wisconsin. Previously, she was director of office operations for Children's Medical Group in Milwaukee. Additionally, she has served in health information management and coordination positions in a variety of healthcare settings. In her volunteer role, Ms. Kuehn has served as secretary and chair of the Ambulatory Care Section of AHIMA and the chair of several national committees. She was a member of the AHIMA Board of Directors for 2005–2007 and is currently a member of the Board of Directors of the AHIMA Foundation. Moreover, she has been active as a presenter at numerous meetings and seminars in the field of physician office management, coding, and reimbursement. Previous AHIMA publications include *Procedural Coding and Reimbursement for Physician Services, A Practical Approach to Analyzing Healthcare Data, Effective Management of Coding Services*, which she edited with Lou Ann Schraffenberger, *Documentation and Reimbursement for Physician Offices,* which she coauthored with LaVonne Wieland, and *The Learning Guide for Ambulatory Care.* Ms. Kuehn has been the recipient of the AHIMA Educator-Practitioner Award and the Wisconsin Health Information Management Association Distinguished Member Award. She holds an MS in health services administration and a BS in medical record administration, is a certified coding specialist–physician-based, and is a Fellow of the American Health Information Management Association.

Preface

Welcome to the pages of this comprehensive *Exam Preparation* manual designed to assist you in taking the certified coding specialist–physician-based (CCS–P) exam. To become a physician-based coder, proficiency in assigning numeric codes for each diagnosis and procedure, in-depth knowledge of the Current Procedural Terminology (CPT®) coding system, and familiarity with the International Classification of Diseases, Ninth Revision, Clinical Modification (ICD-9-CM) and Healthcare Common Procedure Coding System (HCPCS) level II coding systems must be in place. This manual will help you identify less competent areas for further study. However, if at this point in your endeavor, this knowledge base is not as solidly understood as it should be, it is advisable to obtain for study, copies of the following AHIMA publications:

> *ICD-9-CM Diagnostic Coding and Reimbursement for Physician Services*, 2010 Edition (Hazelwood and Venable)

> *Procedural Coding and Reimbursement for Physician Services: Applying Current Procedural Terminology and HCPCS*, 2010 Edition (Kuehn)

Other AHIMA publications cover topics such as health information documentation, data integrity and quality, and additional key areas of expertise required by the coder in the physician practice (available at AHIMA's online bookstore: ahimastore.org).

To fully prepare for the CCS–P exam, consult AHIMA's *Certification Web site (ahima.org/ certification)* to check eligibility requirements, download and submit an exam application, see sample test questions, and find out more about exam day procedures. The site also provides a list of study resources.

The CCS–P exam assesses mastery-level knowledge or proficiency in coding rather than entry-level skills. This certification exam is based on an explicit set of competencies that have been determined by job analysis of coders in physician-based practices. Those competencies are subdivided into domains and tasks that include, in particular, health information documentation, ICD-9-CM diagnosis coding, CPT and HCPCS II coding, as well as reimbursement, data quality and analysis, information and communication technologies, and compliance and regulatory issues. Thorough preparation for taking the CCS–P exam requires that you have already successfully encountered questions in each of these domains. This *Exam Preparation* manual not only provides questions in each of these domains, questions are also designed to align with the formatting and the cognitive levels addressed by questions in part I of the exam: four-option, multiple choice questions written at three cognitive levels: recall, application, and analysis. Part II of the exam requires performance of diagnostic (ICD-9-CM) coding in all specialties and procedural (CPT and HCPCS level II) coding for physician services. A CD-ROM of study questions and practice exams also accompanies this book.

Clearly, the best preparation for the exam is your education. We offer this manual as your guide to success on the CCS–P exam. We have used our collective expertise to compile questions that are aligned to the content areas currently featured in exam questions. The variety of questions ensures the reader of experience with all approaches.

Congratulations! You've chosen to earn credentials in what is forecast to be a favorable professional field. Get ready to study.

About the CD-ROM

The CD-ROM accompanying this book contains 60 multiple choice practice questions and eight practice cases to get you started along with three 60-question multiple choice practice exams that can be run in practice mode or exam simulation mode.

To install the practice exams on your computer:

1. Insert the CD-ROM in your computer's CD/DVD drive.
2. Double-click the .exe file.
3. When asked if you would like to extract files from this archive, select Yes.
4. Accept the license agreement.
5. If offered an installation path, choose the default path suggested.
6. A message will appear stating that the files have been successfully extracted.
7. The Setup Wizard will open.
8. Follow on-screen instructions through setup and install.

Windows Vista users must right-click the .exe file icon and select Run as Administrator.

Minimum system requirements: Intel Pentium II 450MHz or faster processor (or equivalent) with 128MB of RAM running Microsoft Windows 2000, XP, or Vista.

The exam simulations are written for a Microsoft Windows environment. To run the test simulations on a Macintosh, you will need to simulate a Windows environment using additional software for a Mac, such as Apple's Bootcamp. AHIMA cannot guarantee this CD will run on a Mac.

This software product is designed to work on Windows 2000, XP, and Vista. Under most circumstances, installation will be easy. To begin the installation, double-click the Program icon.

Windows Vista users may get an error message on installation. Windows Vista users should right-click the .exe file icon and select Run as Administrator. The program should then extract and install. However, in some controlled environments (such as corporate environments where users are locked down), the process gets a bit more complex. As part of the installation process, some .dll and .ocx files are silently registered into the system registry. This process requires administrative rights, and in some cases, the end user may need to have his or her privileges elevated to install the software. Administrative rights are not needed to actually use the software.

In **Windows Vista**, users without administrative rights will automatically be prompted for the administrative password during the installation. If the user does not have administrative rights, the application, and the shortcut to the application, will not be created on their account—but instead on the administrative user's account. This is obviously not the desired result, but is a consequence of the way Windows Vista works.

How to Use This Book and CD

The CCS–P practice questions and practice exams in this book and on the accompanying CD-ROM test knowledge of content pertaining to the CCS–P competencies published by AHIMA. The multiple choice practice questions and practice exams in this book and CD-ROM are presented in a similar format to those that might be found on the CCS–P exam.

This book contains 60 practice multiple choice questions and eight practice medical cases along with three practice exams (60 multiple choice questions and 16 medical cases each). Because each question is identified by a CCS–P domain, you will be able to determine whether you need knowledge or skill building in particular areas of the exam competencies. Most questions provide a reference for the correct answer. Pursuing these references will help you build your knowledge and skills in specific domains.

To most effectively use this book, work through all the practice questions first. This will help you identify areas in which you may need further preparation. For the questions that you answer incorrectly, read the associated references to help refresh your knowledge. After going through the practice questions, take one of the practice exams. Again, for the questions that you answer incorrectly, refresh your knowledge by reading the associated references. Retake the practice questions and exams as many times as you like.

The CD-ROM includes all the multiple choice questions from the book. Each of the three practice exams on CD can be run in practice mode, which allows you to work at your own pace, or exam mode, which simulates the timed exam experience. The practice questions and practice exams on CD can be set to be presented in random order, or you may choose to go through the questions in sequential order by domain. You may also choose to practice or test your skills on specific domains. For example, if you would like to build your skills in domain 3, you may choose only domain 3 questions for a given practice session.

About the CCS-P Exam

The CCS–P is a coding practitioner with expertise in physician-based settings such as physician offices, group practices, multispecialty clinics, or specialty centers. This coding practitioner reviews patients' records and assigns numeric codes for each diagnosis and procedure. To perform this task, an individual must possess in-depth knowledge of the CPT coding system and familiarity with the ICD-9-CM and HCPCS level II coding systems. The CCS–P is also expert in health information documentation, data integrity, and quality. Because patients' coded data are submitted to insurance companies or the government for expense reimbursement, the CCS–P plays a critical role in the health provider's business operation. What's more, the employment outlook for this coding specialty looks highly favorable with the growth of managed care and the movement of health services delivery beyond the hospital.

The CCS–P certification exam assesses mastery or proficiency in coding rather than entry-level skills. If you perform coding in a doctor's office, clinic, or similar setting, you should consider obtaining the CCS–P certification to attest your ability.

The multiple choice items on the CCS–P exam are designed to test three different cognitive abilities: recall, application, and analysis. These levels represent an organized way to identify the performance that practitioners will utilize on the job. An explanation of the three cognitive levels is provided here:

Cognitive Level	Purpose	Performance Required
Recall (RE)	Primarily measuring memory	Identify terms, specific facts, methods, procedures, basic concepts, basic theories, principles, and processes
Application (AP)	To measure simple interpretation of limited data	Apply concepts and principles to new situations; recognize relationships among data; apply laws and theories to practical situations; calculate solutions to mathematical problems; interpret charts and translate graphic data; classify items; interpret information
Analysis (AN)	To measure the application of knowledge to solving a specific problem and the assembly of various elements into a meaningful whole	Select an appropriate solution for responsive action; revise policy, procedure, or plan; evaluate a solution, case scenario, report, or plan; compare solutions, plans, ideas, or aspects of a problem; evaluate information or a situation; perform multiple calculations to arrive at one answer

Exam Competency Statements

A CCS–P certification exam is based on an explicit set of competencies. These competencies were determined by job analysis surveys of physician-based coders. Exams test only content pertaining to the following competencies:

Domain 1: Health Information Documentation (18 percent)

1. Locate appropriate source documents within the health record for coding or data collection.

2. Interpret health record documentation using knowledge of anatomy, physiology, clinical disease processes, pharmacology, and medical terminology to identify codeable diagnoses and/or procedures.

3. Determine when additional clinical documentation is needed to assign and/or validate the diagnosis and/or procedure code(s).

4. Consult with/query physicians and/or non-physician practitioners when additional information is needed for coding and/or to clarify conflicting or ambiguous information.

5. Consult clinical reference materials to enable interpretation of health information documentation.

6. Determine those elements of the documentation that are extraneous or unnecessary for coding purposes.

Domain 2: ICD-9-CM Diagnosis Coding (24 percent)

1. Apply ICD-9-CM conventions, formats, instructional notations, tables, and definitions to select diagnoses, conditions, problems, or other reasons for the encounter.

2. Assign ICD-9-CM code by applying Diagnostic Coding and Reporting Guidelines for Outpatient Services (Hospital-based and Physician Office).

3. Consult AHA *Coding Clinic* to assist in proper assignment of diagnostic codes.

Domain 3: CPT and HCPCS II Coding (24 percent)

1. Apply CPT guidelines, format, and instructional notes to select services, procedures, and supplies that require coding.

2. Assign CPT code(s) for procedures and/or services rendered during the encounter:
   a. Evaluation and Management (E/M) services
   b. Anesthesia
   c. Surgery
   d. Radiology
   e. Pathology and Laboratory
   f. Medicine
   g. Category III

3. Apply HCPCS II guidelines and instructional notes to select services, procedures, drugs, and supplies that require coding.

4. Assign HCPCS II codes for services, procedures, drugs, and/or supplies provided.

5. Append modifiers to CPT and/or HCPCS II codes when applicable.

Domain 4: Reimbursement (8 percent)

1. Create and maintain encounter form or charge tickets and/or electronic equivalents.
2. Apply bundling and unbundling guidelines (for example, National Correct Coding Initiative [NCCI]).
3. Apply reimbursement methodologies for billing and/or reporting (for example, OIG, CMS, *Federal Register*).
4. Link diagnosis code to the associated procedure code for billing or reporting.
5. Identify, post, and submit charges for healthcare services based on documentation and payer guidelines.
6. Evaluate payer remittance or payment (for example, RA, EOB, EOMB) reports for reimbursement and/or denials.
7. Process claim denials and/or appeals.

Domain 5: Data Quality and Analysis (10 percent)

1. Validate accuracy and completeness of coded data by comparing the documentation to the encounter form or electronic equivalent.
2. Assess the quality of coding and billing using generated reports.
3. Verify the accuracy and completeness of the data on the claim.
4. Conduct coding and billing audits for compliance and trending.
5. Educate healthcare providers and/or staff regarding reimbursement methodologies, documentation rules, and regulations related to coding.

Domain 6: Information and Communication Technologies (6 percent)

1. Use computer systems to ensure data collection, storage, analysis, and reporting of information.
2. Use common software applications (for example, word processing, spreadsheets, email, encoders) in the execution of work processes.

Domain 7: Compliance and Regulatory Issues (10 percent)

1. Apply policies and procedures for access to and disclosure of personal health information.
2. Release patient-specific data to authorized individuals.
3. Apply AHIMA Code of Ethics and Standards of Ethical Coding.
4. Recognize/report privacy issues/problems.
5. Protect data integrity and validity using software or hardware technology.
6. Participate in the development of coding policies to ensure compliance with official coding rules and guidelines.
7. Evaluate the accuracy and completeness of the patient record as defined by organizational policy and external regulations and standards (for example, signature, teaching physician rules, physician assistant [PA] co-sign requirements).
8. Recognize/report compliance concerns/findings.

Exam Specifications

Part I: Multiple Choice consists of 60 four-option multiple choice items.

Part II: Medical Record Coding requires you to perform diagnostic (ICD-9-CM) and procedural (CPT and HCPCS level II) coding for physician services. A total of 16 records from the hospital, emergency room, operating room, and physician office/clinic settings are used:

- 6 cases from the E/M chapter of CPT

- 6 cases from the Surgery chapter of CPT

- 3 cases from the Medicine chapter of CPT

- 1 additional case chosen from the remaining chapters of the CPT book and HCPCS level II

The total testing time for the exam is 4 hours. You cannot return to part I after beginning part II of the exam.

Time Allotted	Activity
20 minutes	Tutorial (not counted as part of the 4-hour exam)
90 minutes	Part I: Multiple choice
10 minutes	Mandatory break (not counted as part of the 4-hour exam). Retrieve codebooks and collect part II CCS–P Exam booklets from the test center administrator.
150 minutes	Part II: Medical record cases

Procedures for Coding Part II of the CCS–P Exam

1. Apply ICD-9-CM instructional notations and conventions and current approved "Basic Coding Guidelines for Outpatient Services" and "Diagnostic Coding and Reporting Requirements for Physician Billing" (*Coding Clinic* for ICD-9-CM, Fourth Quarter, 1995), to select diagnoses, conditions, problems, or other reasons for care that require ICD-9-CM coding in a physician-based encounter/visit either in a physician's office, clinic, outpatient area, emergency room, ambulatory surgery, or other ambulatory care setting. Code for professional services only.

2. Sequencing is not required for the diagnoses or procedures.

3. Do not assign modifiers.

4. Apply the following directions to assign codes to secondary diagnoses:

    a. Chronic diseases treated on an ongoing basis may be coded and reported as many times as the patient is receiving treatment and care for the condition(s).

    b. Code all documented conditions that coexist at the time of the encounter/visit and that require or affect patient care, treatment, or management.

    c. Conditions previously treated and no longer existing are not coded.

5. Code for the professional services only and only for the physician designated on the cover sheet for each individual case.

6. Assign CPT and/or HCPCS Level II codes for all appropriate services.

7. Assign CPT codes for anesthetic procedures listed in the anesthesia section only if indicated on the case cover sheet.

8. Assign CPT codes for medical services/procedures based on current CPT guidelines.

9. Confirm Evaluation and Management (E/M) codes based on the information provided in the box for each case. *For the purposes of this examination, do not challenge the level of key components chosen. You will not be expected to assign the level of history, examinations, and medical decision-making.*

10. Assign CPT codes for radiology and pathology/laboratory procedures listed in the radiology and pathology/laboratory sections only when applicable.

11. Assign CPT codes from the medicine section based on current CPT guidelines.

12. Assign HCPCS Level II National (alphanumeric) codes, as appropriate.

13. Do not assign ICD-9-CM E-codes.

14. Do not assign ICD-9-CM Morphology codes (M-codes).

15. Do not assign ICD-9-CM, Volume 3, procedure codes.

16. Do not assign Category II or Category III CPT codes.

Exam Strategy and Scoring

The CCS–P exam is designed to test accuracy rate and efficiency level of physician-based coding for all specialties. Candidates should pace themselves throughout the examination.

Up to four ICD-9-CM diagnosis and six CPT and/or HCPCS level II procedural codes are to be entered in the spaces provided for the medical records. Medical record coding answers may have fewer codes than the number of spaces provided. Code what is essential, but do not overcode. Points will be deducted for incorrect codes and failure to list a required code. Record only the required digits of the codes; do not fill any blank spaces with zeros or other characters.

Sequencing of diagnoses and operative procedures is not considered in scoring part II of the exam. Points are deducted for inappropriate codes. Follow the procedures listed earlier in the Procedures for Coding Part II of the CCS–P Exam section. These procedures will also be supplied with each section of part II of the exam. Remember that the test will be scored using these procedures. Do not use facility, regional, or insurance standards that differ from the exam procedures.

Because of the lack of standardization in the payer communities across the United States, use of modifiers and linking diagnoses to procedures are tested in part I of the exam only. In order to pass the exam, candidates must meet or exceed the passing scores for both part I and part II of the exam.

What Books to Bring

For exams scheduled on **June 2, 2010 and after** please make sure you have the following codebooks when you report to the test center to take your exam.

- *2010 ICD-9-CM Volumes 1 and 2* (Volume 3 is allowed)
- *2010 CPT* (published by the AMA only)
- *2010 HCPCS National Level II* codebook
- Medical dictionary (optional)

For the CCS–P exam, codebooks are used only for part II. A medical dictionary may be referenced only for part II of the exam.

Candidates without the required codebooks will not be permitted to test and will forfeit their application fee. Candidates who do not bring all the required books, or whose books do not have the correct year, will not be allowed to test. For more detailed CCS–P exam information, visit ahima.org/certification.

Practice Questions
Multiple Choice Questions

Domain 1: Health Information Documentation

1. The paper record format in which the entire record is arranged in strict chronological order is called a(n):

    a. Clinical-entry health record

    b. Integrated health record

    c. Source-oriented health record

    d. Problem-oriented health record

2. In ICD-9-CM, which one of the following is not considered a complication of labor and delivery?

    a. Forceps or vacuum extractor delivery without mention of indication

    b. Cephalic or occipital presentation with spontaneous, vaginal delivery

    c. Anal sphincter tear, not associated with third-degree perineal laceration

    d. Trauma to perineum and vulva during delivery

3. Sometimes referred to as a "superbug," this organism is a major cause of hospital-acquired infection:

    a. Friedlander's bacillus

    b. Pseudomonas

    c. Methicillin-resistant staphylococcus aureus

    d. Coxsackie virus

4. Which of the following is considered a prion disease, a family of rare progressive neuro-degenerative disorders?

    a. Creutzfeldt-Jakob disease

    b. ECHO virus

    c. Cat-scratch disease

    d. Asymptomatic neurosyphilis

5. The coder notes that the physician has prescribed Synthroid for the patient. The coder might find which of the following on the patient's problem list?

   a. Acromegaly

   b. Hypothyroidism

   c. Dwarfism

   d. Cushing's disease

6. A male patient is seen by the physician and diagnosed with pneumonia. The doctor took cultures to try to determine which organism was causing the pneumonia. Which of the following organisms would alert the coder to code it as a gram-negative pneumonia?

   a. Staphylococcus

   b. Clostridium

   c. Klebsiella

   d. Streptococcus

7. Which of the following data elements is needed to accurately assign a CPT preventive medicine code?

   a. Time spent with the patient

   b. Age of the patient

   c. History, examination, and medical decision making

   d. Place of service

8. The physician visits his patient in the hospital and indicates that the patient has diabetes. Insulin is prescribed for and given to the patient. The coding professional should do which of the following?

   a. Assign a code for Type I diabetes mellitus because insulin was given

   b. Assign a code for Type II or unspecified diabetes mellitus because insulin was given

   c. Assign a code for Type II uncontrolled diabetes mellitus

   d. Query the physician to determine which type of diabetes mellitus the patient has

9. Documentation in the health record that relates to the patient's diagnoses and treatment is considered what type of data?

   a. Demographic

   b. Clinical

   c. Financial

   d. Personal

10. The clinical statement, "sections contain oral epithelium with underlying glandular tissue that has both serous and acinar cells" would be documented on which record form?

   a. Physical examination

   b. Operative report

   c. Pathology report

   d. Discharge summary

Domain 2: ICD-9-CM Diagnosis Coding

11. The patient is seen in the Emergency Department with acute lumbar pain. The ED physician documents possible kidney stones and orders an x-ray. The radiologist documents bilateral nephrolithiasis. The coder would assign a code for which of the following conditions:

    a. Acute lumbar pain

    b. Bilateral nephrolithiasis

    c. Possible kidney stones

    d. Abnormal x-ray findings

12. Of the following ICD-9-CM codes, which one can serve as a "stand-alone" code?

    a. V30.00: Single liveborn birth, born in hospital, delivered without mention of Cesarean section

    b. M8070/3: Squamous cell carcinoma

    c. V27.0: Outcome of delivery, single liveborn

    d. E910.4: Accidental drowning and submersion in bathtub

13. A fetal death is defined as a:

    a. Death of a fetus of less than 500 g

    b. Death of a fetus of 20 or more weeks of gestation

    c. Death of a fetus as defined by the physician

    d. Death of a fetus where state law determines weight and weeks of gestation.

14. Using the illustration below from the Table of Drugs and Chemicals in the ICD-9-CM codebook, which E code would a coder select to indicate the external cause for a diagnosis of "Excessive drowsiness due to intentional overdose of Periactin"?

Substance	Poisoning	External Cause (E Code)				
		Accident	Therapeutic Use	Suicide Attempt	Assault	Undetermined
Periactin	963.0	E858.1	E933.0	E950.4	962.0	E980.4

    a. E858.1

    b. E980.4

    c. E950.4

    d. E933.0

15. Using the illustration below from the Table of Drugs and Chemicals in the ICD-9-CM codebook, which E code would a coder select to indicate the external cause for a diagnosis of "Excessive drowsiness due to accidental overdose of Periactin?"

		External Cause (E Code)				
Substance	Poisoning	Accident	Therapeutic Use	Suicide Attempt	Assault	Undetermined
Periactin	963.0	E858.1	E933.0	E950.4	962.0	E980.4

   a. E858.1

   b. E980.4

   c. E950.4

   d. E933.0

16. A "missed abortion" refers to:

   a. Fetal death prior to 20 weeks of gestation

   b. Fetal death prior to actual delivery date

   c. Fetal death prior to completion of 22 weeks of gestation

   d. Fetal death prior to 15 weeks of gestation

17. A diagnosis of elevated blood pressure reading, without a diagnosis of hypertension is assigned code:

   a. 997.91

   b. Code from categories 401–405

   c. 796.2

   d. Code from category 642

18. A female infant was born in the hospital at term and at a normal birth weight. It was a vaginal delivery with a vertex presentation. In the hours after birth, jaundice was noted and eventually a diagnosis of erythroblastosis fetalis due to an ABO incompatibility was made. How would this condition be coded?

V30.00	Single liveborn, born in hospital
773.0	Hemolytic disease due to RH isoimmunization
773.1	Hemolytic disease due to ABO immunization
773.2	Hemolytic disease due to other and unspecified isoimmunization
774.1	Perinatal jaundice and other excessive hemolysis

   a. V30.00; 773.0

   b. V30.00; 773.1

   c. V30.00; 774.1

   d. V30.00; 773.2

19. What is the correct code assignment for an intrauterine pregnancy, term, delivered, right occipitoanterior, liveborn female infant; second-degree lacerations of the perineum?

> 664.11 Second-degree perineal laceration, delivered, with or without mention of antepartum condition
>
> 664.21 Third-degree perineal laceration, delivered, with or without mention of antepartum condition
>
> V27.0 Outcome of delivery, single liveborn
>
> V27.9 Outcome of delivery, unspecified outcome of delivery

    a. 664.11; V27.0

    b. V27.0; 664.21

    c. 664.11; V27.9

    d. 664.21; V27.9

20. A patient visits his physician's office and indicates that he has left arm paralysis due to a case of poliomyelitis that he suffered as a young child. What diagnosis codes would be assigned for this diagnosis?

> 045.9 Acute poliomyelitis, unspecified, poliovirus unspecified type
>
> 138 Late effects of acute poliomyelitis
>
> 342.9 Hemiplegia and hemiparesis, unspecified
>
> 344.40 Monoplegia of upper limb affecting unspecified side
>
> 344.41 Monoplegia of upper limb affecting dominant side
>
> 344.42 Monoplegia of upper limb affecting nondominant side

    a. 344.40; 138

    b. 138; 344.42

    c. 342.9; 045.9

    d. 138; 344.40

21. The physician sees a patient in the hospital with a diagnosis of "metastasis to the brain admitted in a comatose state." In ICD-9-CM, how would this diagnosis be coded?

    a. Code only the brain metastasis (198.3)

    b. Code only the unknown primary site (199.1)

    c. Code the metastasis (198.3) followed by a code for the coma (780.01)

    d. Code only the coma (780.01)

22. What ICD-9-CM code is used to determine "contraceptive sterilization?"

    a. V25.2, sterilization

    b. Underlying medical condition

    c. Code for the incidental pregnancy

    d. Underlying psychological condition

Domain 3: CPT and HCPCS II Coding

23. When CPT codes have resequenced (appear out of the normal order), the code is preceded by which of the following symbols?

    a. "▲"

    b. "○"

    c. "+"

    d. "●"

24. A two-month-old baby presents to the Emergency Department with a high fever. The ED physician performs a detailed history, a detailed examination, and uses high-level medical decision making. The physician also performs a lumbar puncture to remove cerebrospinal fluid sample for culture. How are the ED physician's services coded?

99284	Emergency Department visit for the evaluation and management of a patient, which requires these 3 key components: A detailed history; a detailed examination; and medical decision making of moderate complexity.
99285	Emergency Department visit for the evaluation and management of a patient, which requires these 3 key components: A comprehensive history; a comprehensive examination; and medical decision making of high complexity.
62270	Spinal puncture, lumbar, diagnostic
62272	Spinal puncture, therapeutic, for drainage of cerebrospinal fluid (by needle or catheter)
–25	Significant, separately identifiable Evaluation and Management Service by the same physician on the same day of the procedure or other service.

    a. 99284–25, 62270

    b. 99285–25, 62270

    c. 99284–25, 62272

    d. 99285–25, 62272

25. The physician removes an autograft of iliac crest bone to be used as crushed bone during a lumbar arthrodesis procedure. How is this coded?

    a. 20900: Bone graft, any donor area; minor small (eg, dowel or button)

    b. 20902: Bone graft, any donor area; major or large

    c. 20936: Autograft for spine surgery only (includes harvesting the graft); local (eg, ribs, spinous process, or laminar fragments) obtained from same incision (List separately in addition to code for primary procedure.)

    d. 20937: Autograft for spine surgery only (includes harvesting the graft); morselized (through separate skin or fascial incision) (List separately in addition to code for primary procedure.)

26. The physician treats a patient who has osteomyelitis of the left shoulder blade following a past injury. A piece of dead bone is removed from the body of the shoulder blade and the physician removes surrounding bone to return the shoulder blade to its natural contour. How is this coded?

> 23140 Excision or curettage of bone cyst or benign tumor of clavicle or scapula
>
> 23170 Sequestrectomy (eg, for osteomyelitis or bone abscess), clavicle
>
> 23172 Sequestrectomy (eg, for osteomyelitis or bone abscess), scapula
>
> 23180 Partial excision (craterization, saucerization, or disphysectomy) bone (eg, osteomyelitis), clavicle
>
> 23182 Partial excision (craterization, saucerization, or disphysectomy) bone (eg, osteomyelitis), scapula
>
> 23190 Ostectomy of scapula, partical (eg, superior medial angle)

   a. 23170–LT, 23140–51–LT

   b. 23172–LT, 23140–51–LT

   c. 23172–LT, 23182–51–LT

   d. 23190–LT, 23180–51–LT

27. The physician curettes three lesions off the patient's back. The lesions are keratotic and measure 0.5 cm each. How is this service coded?

> 11400 Excision, benign lesion including margins, except skin tag (unless listed elsewhere), trunk, arms, or legs; excised diameter 0.5 cm or less
>
> 11402   excised diameter 1.1 to 2.0 cm
>
> 17000 Destruction (eg, laser surgery, electrosurgery, cryosurgery, chemosurgery, surgical curettement), premalignant lesions (eg, actinic keratoses); first lesion
>
> 17003   second through 14 lesions, each (List separately in addition to code for first lesion)

   a. 11400, 11400–51, 11400–51

   b. 11402

   c. 17000

   d. 17000, 17003, 17003

28. A 32-year-old female patient presents to the urgent care center after eating a fish sandwich, stating that she has a stabbing pain in the throat as she swallows or clears her throat. The physician examines her larynx using a mirror, locates a small fish bone lodged in the muscular wall of the larynx and removes it using a long-nosed forceps. How are these services coded?

> 31505 Laryngoscopy, indirect; diagnostic (separate procedure)
>
> 31511   with removal of foreign body
>
> 31515 Laryngoscopy direct, with or without tracheoscopy; for aspiration
>
> 31530 Laryngoscopy, direct, operative, with foreign body removal

    a. 31511

    b. 31505, 31511–51

    c. 31515

    d. 31530

29. The physician performs therapeutic injections of both the patient's facet joints at T12–L1 and L1–L2, using fluoroscopic guidance. How is this coded?

> 64490 Injection, diagnostic or therapeutic agent, paravertebral facet (zygopophyseal) joint (or nerves innervating that joint) with image guidance (fluoroscopy or CT), cervical or thoracic; single level
>
> 64493 Injection, diagnostic or therapeutic agent, paravertebral facet (zygopophyseal) joint (or nerves innervating that joint) with image guidance (fluoroscopy or CT), lumbar or sacral; single level
>
> 64494   second level (List separately in addition to code for primary procedure)
>
> 64495   third and any additional level(s) (List separately in addition to code for primary procedure)
>
> –50   Bilateral procedure

    a. 64493-50, 64494–50

    b. 64490-50, 64494–50

    c. 64493, 64493

    d. 64495

30. The physician performs a median sternotomy and places the patient on cardiopulmonary bypass to repair the patient's aortopulmonary window, or a connection between the aorta and pulmonary artery just above the semilunar valves. The physician opens the pulmonary artery and locates the window, closing it with a Dacron fabric patch. The patient is taken off bypass and the sternal incision is closed. How is this procedure coded?

    a. 33645: Direct or patch closure, sinus venosus, with or without anomalous pulmonary venous drainage

    b. 33813: Obliteration of aortopulmonary septal defect; without cardiopulmonary bypass

    c. 33814: Obliteration of aortopulmonary septal defect; with cardiopulmonary bypass

    d. 33917: Repair of pulmonary artery stenosis by reconstruction with patch or graft

31. The physician débrides and dresses second degree burns on the patient's entire left leg and foot. How is this coded?

    a. 11000: Débridement of extensive eczematous or infected skin; up to 10% of body surface

    b. 11040: Débridement; skin, partial thickness

    c. 16025: Dressings and/or débridement of partial-thickness burns, initial or subsequent; medium (eg, whole face or whole extremity, or 5% to 10% total body surface area)

    d. 16030: Dressings and/or débridement of partial-thickness burns, initial or subsequent; large (eg, more than 1 extremity, or greater than 10% total body surface area)

32. The patient undergoes a CT colonography using contrast material to diagnose and stage colon cancer. How is this procedure coded?

    a. 45378: Colonoscopy, flexible, proximal to splenic flexure; diagnostic, with or without collection of specimen(s) by brushing or washing, with or without colon decompression (separate procedure)

    b. 74262: Computed tomographic (CT) colonography, diagnostic, including image postprocessing; with contrast images, if performed

    c. 74363: Computer tomographic (CT) colonography, screening, including image postprocessing

    d. 91299: Unlisted diagnostic gastroenterology procedure

33. The physician orders the following blood tests, which are performed together at the office: Carbon dioxide, Chloride, Potassium, Sodium. How are these tests coded?

80051	Electrolyte panel: Carbon dioxide; Chloride; Potassium; Sodium
80053	Comprehensive metabolic panel: Albumin; Bilirubin, total; Calcium, total; Carbon dioxide; Chloride; Creatinine; Glucose; Phosphatase, alkaline; Potassium; Protein, total; Sodium; ALT/SGPT; AST/SGOT; Urea nitrogen
82374	Carbon dioxide (bicarbonate)
82435	Chloride; blood
82436	urine
84132	Potassium; serum, plasma or whole blood
84133	urine
84295	Sodium; serum, plasma or whole blood
84302	other source

    a. 82374, 82435, 84132, 84295

    b. 82374, 82436, 84133, 84302

    c. 80051

    d. 80053

34. During a 50-minute follow-up office visit, the physician provides psychotherapy and spends 5 minutes reviewing medications and adjusting dosages. How is this service coded?

90807	Individual psychotherapy, insight oriented, behavior modifying and/or supportive, in an office or outpatient facility, approximately 45 to 50 minutes face-to-face with the patient; with medical evaluation and management services
90862	Pharmacologic management, including prescription, use, and review of medication with no more than minimal medical psychotherapy
99215	Office or other outpatient visit for the evaluation and management of an established patient, which requires at least 2 of these 3 key components: A comprehensive history; comprehensive examination; medical decision making of high complexity. Physicians typically spend 40 minutes face-to-face with the patient and/or family.
99354	Prolonged physician service in the office or other outpatient setting requiring direct (face-to-face) patient contact beyond the usual service; first hour (List separately in addition to code for office or other outpatient Evaluation and Management service)

a. 99215

b. 99215, 99354

c. 90807

d. 90807, 90862

35. After completion of allergy testing, the allergist prepares and provides allergenic extracts in 20 single-dose vials to begin desensitization. These vials are sent to the patient's primary care physician, who will administer the injections according to the prescribed schedule. How are the services of the allergist coded?

95117	Professional services for allergen immunotherapy not including provision of allergenic extracts; 2 or more injections
95144	Professional services for the supervision of preparation and provision of antigens for allergen immunotherapy, single dose vial(s) (specify number of vials)
95165	Professional services for the supervision of preparation and provision of antigens for allergen immunotherapy; single or multiple antigens (specify number of doses)
95199	Unlisted allergy/clinical immunologic service or procedure

a. 95117 ×10

b. 95144 ×20

c. 95165 ×20

d. 95199

36. A 9-year-old boy is seen in the Emergency Department and receives 560 units of rabies immune globulin and rabies vaccine as intramuscular injections after being bitten by a squirrel that exhibited signs of being infected. The documentation contains an expanded problem focused history, a detailed examination and high-level medical decision making. How are these services coded?

99283	Emergency Department visit with an expanded problem focused history, an expanded problem focused examination, and medical decision making of moderate complexity
99284	Emergency Department visit with a detailed history, a detailed examination, and medical decision making of moderate complexity
99285	Emergency Department visit with a comprehensive history, a comprehensive examination, and medical decision making of high complexity
90375	Rabies immune globulin (RIg), human, for intramuscular and/or subcutaneous use
90471	Immunization administration (includes percutaneous, intradermal, subcutaneous, or intramuscular injections); 1 vaccine (single or combination vaccine/toxoid)
90675	Rabies vaccine, for intramuscular use
90676	Rabies vaccine, for intradermal use
96372	Therapeutic, prophylactic, or diagnostic injection (specify substance or drug); subcutaneous or intramuscular

   a. 99283, 90376, 90675
   b. 99283, 90375, 90675, 90471, 96372
   c. 99284, 90375 ×560, 90675, 96372 ×2
   d. 99285, 90375, 90676, 90471, 96372

37. The nephrologist performs a needle biopsy of the liver using imaging guidance provided by the radiologist. How are the services of the nephrologist coded?
   a. 10022: Fine needle aspiration, with imaging guidance
   b. 47000: Biopsy of liver, percutaneous
   c. 47100: Biopsy of liver, wedge
   d. 47399: Unlisted procedure, liver

38. A 15-year-old patient with type I diabetes and severe complications of insulin administration undergoes a pancreatic islet cell transplantation from an allogeneic, cross-matched source. The islets are transplanted through an abdominal incision and injected into the portal vein. What is the correct code assignment for this service?
   a. 0141T: Pancreatic islet cell transplantation through portal vein, percutaneous
   b. 0142T: Pancreatic islet cell transplantation through portal vein, open
   c. 48554: Transplantation of pancreatic allograft
   d. 48999: Unlisted procedure, pancreas

39. The patient has L2-3 spinal stenosis. The surgeon removes the lower portion of the L2 spinous process and the upper portion of the L3 spinous process, as well as the inter-spinous ligament to provide access to the space. A spinous process distraction device is then inserted using imaging guidance. How is this service coded?

22102	Partial excision of posterior vertebral component (eg, spinous process, lamina or facet) for intrinsic bony lesion, single vertebral segment, lumbar
22612	Arthrodesis, posterior or posterolateral technique, single level; lumbar (with or without lateral transverse technique)
22841	Internal spinal fixation by wiring of spinous processes (List separately in addition to code for primary procedure)
0171T	Insertion of posterior spinous process distraction device (including necessary removal of bone or ligament for insertion and imaging guidance), lumbar; single level

    a. 22102, 22841

    b. 22612, 22841

    c. 0171T

    d. 22102, 0171T

40. The physician orders and administers 600 mg of IV levofloxacin. How many units of code J1956 would be billed?

J1956	Levofloxacin, 250 mg

    a. 1

    b. 2

    c. 3

    d. 4

41. The patient undergoes a complex cystometrogram with bladder voiding pressure studies at the hospital, completed by their urologist. How does the urologist code for this service?

51726	Complex cystometrogram (ie, calibrated electronic equipment)
51728	Complex cystometrogram (ie, calibrated electronic equipment); with voiding pressure studies (ie, bladder voiding pressure), any technique
51729	Complex cystometrogram (ie, calibrated electronic equipment); with voiding pressure studies (ie, bladder voiding pressure) and urethral pressure profile studies (ie, urethral closure pressure profile), any technique
51798	Measurement of post-voiding residual urine and/or bladder capacity by ultrasound, non-imaging
−26	Professional component

    a. 51726–26

    b. 51728–26

    c. 51729

    d. 51728–26, 51798

Domain 4: Reimbursement

42. Medicare's allowed fee for an in-office procedure is $200. Dr. Smith is a PAR physician and Dr. Jones is a non-PAR physician who does not accept assignment. How much will Dr. Smith and Dr. Jones, respectively, receive from CMS?

    a. $160, $152

    b. $200, $152

    c. $160, $0

    d. $200, $0

43. Medicare's allowed fee for an in-office procedure is $200. Dr. Smith is a PAR physician and Dr. Jones is a non-PAR physician who does not accept assignment. How much will Dr. Smith and Dr. Jones receive, respectively, in total for this procedure?

    a. $200, $200

    b. $160, $152

    c. $200, $218.50

    d. $200, $230

44. When a patient is covered by Medicare, which of the following services will be reimbursed?

    a. General Health laboratory panel

    b. Consultation E/M codes

    c. A preventive medicine service at the start of coverage

    d. Certain transplant services such as pancreas and cornea

45. The physician performs, interprets and reports a 12-lead EKG in the office. Later in the day, the same physician interprets and reports a 64-lead EKG in the heart center at the hospital. Referencing these NCCI Column 1 and Column 2 edits, which code requires a –59 modifier for payment?

Column 1	Column 2
0180T	0179T
0180T	93000
0180T	93005
0180T	93010
0180T	93040
0180T	93041
0180T	93042

  a. 93000: Electrocardiogram, routine ECG with at least 12 leads; with interpretation and report

  b. 93010: Electrocardiogram, routine ECG with at least 12 leads; interpretation and report only

  c. 0178T: Electrocardiogram, 64 leads or greater, with graphic presentation and analysis; with interpretation and report

  d. 0180T: Electrocardiogram, 64 leads or greater, with graphic presentation and analysis; interpretation and report only

46. For FY 2010, the federal government wants to reduce the overall payment to physicians. To incur the least amount of revision, which of the following elements of the RBRVS should CMS reduce?

  a. Practice expense RVU

  b. GPCI

  c. Conversion factor

  d. Work RVU

47. All of the following are cost-sharing provisions of healthcare insurance **except:**

  a. Benefit

  b. Formulary

  c. Copayment

  d. Limitation

Domain 5: Data Quality and Analysis

48. A physician requests that the office manager identify any potentially significant issues in the ICD-9-CM code assignment for the past fiscal year. The best report to review would be the:

    a. Diagnosis distribution report

    b. Service distribution report

    c. Revenue production report

    d. Charge summary report

49. There are several characteristics of data quality. Which of the following is not one of these characteristics?

    a. Consistency

    b. Analysis

    c. Precision

    d. Timeliness

50. A patient covered by Medicare is admitted on the evening of 1-14-2010. The attending physician completes the Initial Hospital Service and submits the following codes to describe the service. What education should take place regarding this claim?

Date	CPT Code	ICD-9-CM Code
1-15-10	99223: Level 3 Initial Hospital Service	820.20: Fracture of neck of femur, pertro-chanteric fracture, closed, unspecified

    a. Level 3 Initial Hospital service codes are frequently the subject of government audits.

    b. The ICD-9-CM code does not appear specific.

    c. Modifier AI (Principle physician of record) was not assigned.

    d. The date of service is incorrect.

Domain 6: Information and Communication Technologies

51. A physician wants to graphically show the increase in numbers of patients he has treated over the last 15 years. Which of the following would best be used to depict this data?

    a. Bar chart

    b. Pie chart

    c. Line graph

    d. Histogram

52. Which of the following is a barrier to effective computer-assisted coding?

    a. Ability of the computer to apply coding rules

    b. Resistance by physicians

    c. Lack of complete clinical documentation

    d. Resistance by coders

53. Storing duplicate data at a distant location is an example of:

    a. Data mapping

    b. Data mining

    c. Data storage for recovery

    d. Data redundancy

54. The _____ is a type of coding that uses software to automatically generate a set of medical codes based on documentation by the healthcare provider.

    a. Natural language processing

    b. Encoder

    c. Automated codebook

    d. Computer-assisted coding

Domain 7: Compliance and Regulatory Issues

55. A legal, written document that specifies patient preferences regarding future healthcare or designates a person to assume authority for the patient is known as a(n):

    a. Court order

    b. Subpoena duces decum

    c. Covered entity

    d. Advance directive

56. Under HIPAA's Privacy and Security Rules, which one of the following is not considered a covered entity?

    a. Healthcare providers

    b. Healthcare clearinghouse

    c. Life insurance company

    d. Health plan

57. HIM coding professionals and the organizations that employ them have the responsibility to not tolerate behavior that adversely affects data quality. Which of the following is an example of behavior that should not be tolerated?

    a. Assign codes to an incomplete record without organizational policies in place to ensure codes are reviewed after the records are complete

    b. Follow up on and monitor identified problems

    c. Evaluate and trend diagnoses and procedures code selections

    d. Report data quality review results to organizational leadership, compliance staff, and the medical staff

58. In a hospital, the Business/Accounting Department has a legitimate access to a patient's health record without the patient's authorization. This statement is based on what HIPAA principle/standard?

    a. Preemption

    b. Minimum necessary

    c. Disclosure accounting

    d. Statute of limitations

59. Minors are generally unable to access, use, or disclose their personal health information. What resource should be cited as to who may legally authorize disclosure of a minor's health record?

    a. Chief information officer for the hospital

    b. Individual state law(s) since HIPAA defers to state law on such matters

    c. Hospital attorney hired by the facility

    d. HIPAA because of the strict rules regarding minors

60. An exception to the required consent requirement for treatment includes a(n):

    a. Implied consent

    b. Informed consent

    c. Physician discretion

    d. Medical emergency

Practice Medical Cases

Practice Cases   CASE 1

PICU PROGRESS NOTE

CHIEF COMPLAINT: Wheezing

HISTORY OF PRESENT ILLNESS: The patient is a 25-month-old boy, transported here yesterday from the community hospital with a history of acute onset of respiratory distress and desaturation on room air. Clinical picture is initially consistent with first episode of wheezing. His respiratory distress has responded to Albuterol, Atrovent, Solumedrol, and Magnesium sulfate. However, he has persistent elevated anion gap that is not well explained.

OVERNIGHT EVENTS: The patient was initially treated with continuous Albuterol at 10 mg/hr, Atrovent q 6 hours, Solumedrol ×6 hours, and he was given one dose of Magnesium sulfate IV for continued respiratory distress, with resulting decrease in tachypnea and improvement in wheezing. However, he showed a persistent metabolic acidosis with an elevated anion gap. Given that metabolic acidosis did not improve after aggressive fluid rehydration, and the anion gap was elevated, a search was carried out for possible etiologies. His initial serum glucose prior to initiation of steroid therapy was 178, and he did begin spilling ketones and glucose in his urine. We therefore elected to treat for possible diabetic ketoacidosis. His hyperglycemia rapidly resolved on Insulin 0.05 units/kg/hour and aggressive fluid and electrolyte replacement. He was quiet from a neurologic standpoint overnight, responding with appropriate distress to multiple blood draws and verbally interacting with parents.

On further history, there is a family history of diabetes type 2 in grandmother. There is no antecedent polyuria or polydypsia. No weight loss. He had been completely well until 3 days prior to admission when he developed URI symptoms which developed into acute respiratory distress yesterday, necessitating ED visit to outside hospital and subsequent transfer here.

PHYSICAL EXAMINATION:

VITAL SIGNS: TEMPERATURE: 37.4, **HEART RATE:** 147-199, **MBP:** 60–95, **R:** 28-52, **OXYGEN SATURATION:** 96–100%, **INPUT:** 1087 **OUTPUT:** 853

GENERAL: Alert, says "No" or "Okay," appears more tired than yesterday's exam on admission, somewhat pale

> **HEENT:** NCAT, TM's mildly red and partially wax impacted, no rhinorrhea, neck supple, no LAD

> **CARDIOVASCULAR:** Tachycardia, regular sinus rhythm, no m/r/g

> **PULMONARY:** Tachypnea, bilateral expiratory wheeze and prolonged expiratory phase, retractions

> **ABDOMEN:** Soft, ND/NT, +BS, no masses or HSM

> **EXTREMITIES:** WWP, symmetrical movements, CFT, 2 sec

> **NEURO:** Somewhat more tired appearing than yesterday but still responds "Okay" to questions, symmetric movements UE and LE b/l, normal muscle bulk and tone, good strength when fighting blood draw today, EOMI, PERRL at 3 mm.

LABS: Serum ketones 10 (elevated), urine glucose 250–800

CXR: Hyperinflation, PBT, no infiltrate

ASSESSMENT: Previously healthy 25-month-old boy with history of rapid onset of acute respiratory distress and wheezing. His pulmonary clinical picture is consistent with first time reactive airway disease exacerbation with good response to typical asthma meds. However, he has persistent elevated anion gap acidosis and treatment for diabetic ketoacidosis is just beginning. Is on step 1 of new diabetes clinical pathway.

PLAN:

1. Diabetes mellitus, type 1, new onset. Follow clinical pathway, advancing diet to clears and assess tolerance. Follow I/Os. Get chem.-8 BID and CBC with lytes q 6 hours. Parents to step 1 education this afternoon.

2. Reactive airway disease, still with tachycardia and slightly tachypneic. Continue to observe as ketoacidosis resolves. Continue albuterol q 4 hrs prn. Transitioned from Solumedrol to Prednisone 2 mg/kg/day and will continue for total of 5-day course. Discontinue Atrovent. Repeat CXR prn for increasing respiratory distress.

3. Social work consult. Patient and parents are from out of state and visiting grandparents here. Mom in particular is quite worried about patient and his ability to complete travel plans to return home. Social work to assist with airline changes.

Answer Sheet

Directions: Be sure to enter all medical record codes in the manner provided in the sample below, paying special attention to the decimal placement for each code. The codes must be typed on the answer sheet in the boxes provided on the computer screen using the keyboard. A decimal point (.) has been provided as a guide for entering each ICD-9-CM code. **You will lose credit if the digits of the codes are correct, but the decimal point has been incorrectly placed.**

CASE 1 DIAGNOSES   **ICD-9-CM**

DX1				.		
DX2				.		
DX3				.		
DX4				.		

CASE 1 PROCEDURES   **CPT/HCPCS**

PR1					
PR2					
PR3					
PR4					
PR5					
PR6					

Practice Cases CASE 2

PROCEDURE NOTE

PREOPERATIVE DIAGNOSIS: Hodgkins, nodular sclerosis   *201.5*

POSTOPERATIVE DIAGNOSIS: Same

PROCEDURE: Bone marrow aspirates   *38270, 99*

Procedure performed in OR under anesthesia. Patient identified and consent obtained.

Bone marrow studies performed today as patient is having a mediport placed by general surgery during same operative session.

38221
11-gauge Jamshidi biopsy needle used. Bone marrow biopsy sample obtained from right posterior iliac crest and sent to pathology.

Tolerated procedure without complications and was handed to surgery team for placement of port.

Answer Sheet

Directions: Be sure to enter all medical record codes in the manner provided in the sample below, paying special attention to the decimal placement for each code. The codes must be typed on the answer sheet in the boxes provided on the computer screen using the keyboard. A decimal point (.) has been provided as a guide for entering each ICD-9-CM code. **You will lose credit if the digits of the codes are correct, but the decimal point has been incorrectly placed.**

CASE 2 DIAGNOSES   **ICD-9-CM**

DX1				.		
DX2				.		
DX3				.		
DX4				.		

CASE 2 PROCEDURES   **CPT/HCPCS**

PR1					
PR2					
PR3					
PR4					
PR5					
PR6					

Practice Cases   CASE 3

REQUESTING PHYSICIAN: ED attending

HISTORY OF PRESENT ILLNESS: The patient is seen in the ED at 8:25 a.m., accompanied by father. The patient is a 5-year-old boy who was in his normal state of health last night at bedtime. His sister woke parents at about 3:30 a.m. this morning because he was crying. He had fallen out of bed, onto the floor and hit his forehead. Father was called to bedroom and observed a 1-minute episode of tonic posturing of arms and legs in extension. Father reports patient was frightened but aware and able to speak during the episode. Father took him to his bed and a similar episode occurred as soon as the patient fell asleep. Father took him to the living room to sit him up and noticed that patient was weak and unable to walk. There were 10 episodes in all, the last one in the car on the way to the hospital. Every attack occurred as the patient fell asleep and these were similar in appearance. He had no further seizures since arriving at the ED at 6 a.m.

He has had no fever and no signs of illness recently. About two years ago, he had 2 episodes of brief posturing during sleep and was seen in the ED here, but had no tests. He was not febrile at that time.

MEDICATIONS:

1. Advair
2. Singulair
3. Albuterol, prn

PAST MEDICAL HISTORY: He has a history of asthma and has been hospitalized once for wheezing. He takes Advair and Singulair and uses Albuterol prn.

DEVELOPMENT: He has had normal motor and language development. He is ready for kindergarten this year.

FAMILY HISTORY: He has two siblings, age 12 and 7, all living with parents. His maternal grandmother takes Dilantin for seizures.

PHYSICAL EXAMINATION:

VITAL SIGNS: WEIGHT: 17.6 **BLOOD PRESSURE:** 122/66 **TEMPERATURE:** 96.6 **HEART RATE:** 110 **RESPIRATORY RATE:** 24

MENTAL STATUS: Alert and cooperative. Normal speech and behavior for age.

CRANIAL NERVES: Pupils are equal and reactive to light. Eye movements are full and symmetrical. Optic fundi are normal. Face movements are full and symmetrical. Tongue and palate appear normal.

MUSCULOSKELETAL: He has normal muscle bulk, tone, and strength. Left handed.

SENSORY: Intact to tickle of his feet

REFLEXES: Tendon reflexes are active and symmetrical. Plantar responses are flexor.

COORDINATION: No tremor on pointing

GAIT: Stable, runs well

OTHER: Non-dysmorphic features. No rash. No birth marks. Auscultation of heart and lungs is normal. No cervical lymphadenopathy. Cranium and spine are normal.

TESTING: EEG today shows normal background activity awake, drowsy, and asleep. There are frequent spikes in the right temporal and left temporal regions, more frequent during sleep.

IMPRESSION: This is a 5-year-old boy with normal growth and development who presents with multiple brief generalized seizures, each occurring at sleep onset. His EEG shows that he has benign temporal lobe epilepsy.

PLAN:

1. Begin Carbamazepine 100 mg BID for one week, then 100/200. Rx given for #90 with 6 refills.
2. Lab for CBC, LFT, Carbamazepine level in 4 weeks.
3. Follow-up in Neurology Clinic in 6 weeks.
4. Patient/family education: Written information about epilepsy and carbamazepine.

TIME SPENT: 45 minutes

OUTPATIENT ELECTROENCEPHALOGRAM REPORT

The patient is a 5-year-old boy who has had several episodes of shaking without loss of responsiveness this morning.

MEDICATIONS: Advair, Singulair, and Albuterol prn

DESCRIPTION: This is a digital electroencephalogram recorded using the 10–20 Electrode Placement system. The recording was performed following sleep deprivation. The patient is awake, drowsy, and asleep during the recording.

The background activity awake consists of some moderate voltage rhythmic posterior 8 Hz alpha activity. There is much low to moderate voltage generalized 5 to 7 Hz theta activity also present. When he is drowsy, there is much moderate voltage generalized 4 to 6 Hz theta activity present. During sleep vertex sharp waves and central sleep spindles are prominent. There are occasional K-complexes present.

When he is awake, there are occasional moderate voltage spikes present in the temporal regions, both right and left. The spike activity becomes more frequent during drowsiness and sleep.

There is a good symmetrical driving response to intermittent photic stimulation. Hyperventilation produced much moderate to high voltage generalized 3 to 4 Hz delta activity that persisted for longer on the right posteriorly compared to the left.

IMPRESSION: This is an abnormal electroencephalogram. Background activity is normal for age during awake, drowsy, and sleep states. There are occasional spikes present in the right and left temporal lobes during waking that become frequent during drowsiness and sleep. The finding is consistent with multifocal epileptogenic abnormality in the temporal areas. The location of the spikes is consistent with benign temporal epilepsy. Correlation with clinical findings is recommended.

Answer Sheet

Directions: Be sure to enter all medical record codes in the manner provided in the sample below, paying special attention to the decimal placement for each code. The codes must be typed on the answer sheet in the boxes provided on the computer screen using the keyboard. A decimal point (.) has been provided as a guide for entering each ICD-9-CM code. **You will lose credit if the digits of the codes are correct, but the decimal point has been incorrectly placed.**

CASE 3 DIAGNOSES

ICD-9-CM

DX1				.		
DX2				.		
DX3				.		
DX4				.		

CASE 3 PROCEDURES

CPT/HCPCS

PR1					
PR2					
PR3					
PR4					
PR5					
PR6					

Practice Cases   CASE 4

PROCEDURE NOTE

FINDINGS: There was a 1.6 × 1.5-cm congenital defect of the right nasal sidewall that did not involve the alar cartilages. It did extend slightly onto the cheek.

PROCEDURE: After obtaining informed consent, the patient was taken into the operating room and placed in a supine position on the operating table. General anesthesia was induced via endotracheal intubation without difficulty. Approximately 2 mL of 1% lidocaine with 1:100,000 epinephrine was injected into the right conchal bowl and the right postauricular region. The face was prepped and draped in a sterile fashion. A surgical pause was performed to confirm the patient's identity and site of surgery.

A skin incision was made in the conchal bowl on the right-hand side, and a piece of conchal bowl cartilage measuring approximately 1 × 1.5 cm was harvested and placed in saline to be used as a strut along the right lateral sidewall. This incision was closed using 6-0 fast-absorbing gut.

A piece of foil was used to create a template of the defect in the nose. A full-thickness skin graft matching to the shape of a template was harvested from the right postauricular region. The cartilage was then placed along the lateral sidewall and secured in place with a single through-and-through fast-absorbing gut suture. The central portion of the full-thickness skin graft was also secured with a fast-absorbing gut suture to the central portion of the nasal defect. The perimeter of the graft was then sutured to the nose using interrupted 6-0 nylon suture.

Once the graft had been sutured in place, the harvested site in the postauricular region was expanded into an elliptical-shaped defect by removing some skin superior and inferior to the harvest site itself. Undermining was performed primarily in the posterior direction of the skin under the hairline. Minimal undermining was done of the skin anteriorly toward the pinna of the ear. Hemostasis was obtained after the undermining, and this harvest site incision was closed using 4-0 Vicryl and 5-0 nylon. A small pressure dressing was applied to the right side of the nose, and a Glasscock mastoid dressing was placed on the right ear.

The patient was then awakened from the anesthetic, extubated, and transported to the recovery room with stable vital signs and no evidence of stridor.

Answer Sheet

Directions: Be sure to enter all medical record codes in the manner provided in the sample below, paying special attention to the decimal placement for each code. The codes must be typed on the answer sheet in the boxes provided on the computer screen using the keyboard. A decimal point (.) has been provided as a guide for entering each ICD-9-CM code. **You will lose credit if the digits of the codes are correct, but the decimal point has been incorrectly placed.**

CASE 4 DIAGNOSES   **ICD-9-CM**

DX1				.	
DX2				.	
DX3				.	
DX4				.	

CASE 4 PROCEDURES   **CPT/HCPCS**

PR1					
PR2					
PR3					
PR4					
PR5					
PR6					

Practice Cases CASE 5

PSYCHIATRY PROGRESS NOTE

Date: 2/15/XX

Length of Service: 50 minutes

Location: Office

NOTES: The patient has continued to work on "Oceans of Emotions" workbook to help identify and understand her emotions better. Worked on short- and long-term goals—socially, academically, emotionally. She denies any difficulty with school with organization or concentration. She does endorse wanting more friends.

MSE: Alert, casually groomed wearing jeans and fleece; cooperative, good eye contact

Speech: Normal

Thought Process: Linear

Thought Content: Appropriate

Mood: "Fine"

Affect: Somewhat anxious at times

Insight and Judgment: Fair/good

Attention: Fair

Changes to Meds Since Last Visit: None. No side effects reported. Good compliance.

CURRENT MEDS:
Risperdal 1 mg TID
Adderall XR 30 mg q am, Adderall 15 mg at 2 pm
Celexa 5 mg q day
Bactrim for acne

DIAGNOSES:

1. ADHD
2. Reactive adjustment disorder with anxiety

PLAN:

1. Continue current meds
2. Mother met with therapist for family therapy, patient to be scheduled in March
3. Insurance has approved up to 8 more visits

TREATMENT PLAN GOALS:

1. Decrease mood dysregulation
2. Decrease self-injurious behaviors
3. Decrease anxiety
4. Improve socialization
5. Improve self-esteem
6. Improve academic performance

Answer Sheet

Directions: Be sure to enter all medical record codes in the manner provided in the sample below, paying special attention to the decimal placement for each code. The codes must be typed on the answer sheet in the boxes provided on the computer screen using the keyboard. A decimal point (.) has been provided as a guide for entering each ICD-9-CM code. **You will lose credit if the digits of the codes are correct, but the decimal point has been incorrectly placed.**

CASE 5 DIAGNOSES   ICD-9-CM

DX1				.		
DX2				.		
DX3				.		
DX4				.		

CASE 5 PROCEDURES   CPT/HCPCS

PR1					
PR2					
PR3					
PR4					
PR5					
PR6					

Practice Cases

CASE 6

PREOPERATIVE DIAGNOSIS: Right hip labral tear

POSTOPERATIVE DIAGNOSIS: Right hip labral tear

ANESTHESIA: General endotracheal

PROCEDURE: Right hip arthroscopic labral débridement

COMPLICATIONS: None

DRAINS: None

ESTIMATED BLOOD LOSS: Minimal

PROPHYLAXIS: Ancef

OPERATIVE FINDINGS: The patient was noted to have a labral tear in the superior portion of the acetabular labrum with a frayed portion of the labrum hanging down inferiorly. Also noted to have some tearing of the tissue along the pulvinar at the attachment of the ligementum along the acetabular side as well. No articular lesions seen. No loose bodies seen. No other significant findings.

INDICATION FOR PROCEDURE: The patient is a 22-year-old female complaining of right hip pain. MRI confirms evidence of a labral tear. The patient also had a diagnostic injection with relief of pain and requires a right hip arthroscopic labral débridement versus repair. I discussed with the patient all risks, benefit, alternatives, and complications of the procedure including, but not limited to, infection, bleeding, damage to nerves or blood vessels, failure to relieve hip pain, decreased range of motion, reaction to anesthesia, etc. She understands and would like to proceed with operative intervention. All questions were answered. Consent is signed and on the chart prior to the start of the procedure.

PROCEDURE IN DETAIL: After the patient indicated that the right hip was the correct operative site, it was marked in the pre-op holding area by the surgeon. The patient was then taken to the operating room and placed in the supine position on the Chick table with all bony prominences adequately padded. Perineal post was placed. A Foley catheter was placed. The patient was placed in boots bilaterally and traction was applied with the patient's hip in slight abduction and neutral rotation. Fluoroscopic images done by Radiology demonstrated an appropriate distraction. Traction was then let off. The right hip and lower extremity were then prepped and draped in the normal sterile fashion. Traction was applied and time out was called in the room prior to incision. Next using fluoroscopic guidance, a spinal needle was passed at the anterolateral portal staying just anterior to the greater trochanter approximately 2 cm. Spinal needle was easily advanced into the hip joint. Hip articulation with an air arthrogram achieved under fluoroscopy. Next, Nitinol wire was passed through this needle into the hip joint and after making an incision with an 11 blade and having infiltrated the joint with saline with good return, a trocar was then advanced into the hip articulation with a 5.5 cannula placed. Arthroscope was then placed and diagnostic arthroscopy was performed with the above mentioned findings. Next, at the intersection of the greater trochanter and anterior superior iliac spine at the anterior portal needle localization under direct visualization was done, noting good placement within the hip joint. Through a percutaneous incision once again, another 5.5 cannula was placed and a soft tissue shaver and electrocautery were then used to débride the frayed tissue at the pulvinar as well as address the superior labral tear. This was probed and noted to have a flap tear particularly on the undersurface. Using both the flexible probe cautery as well as a curve and straight meniscal shaver through these cannulas by alternating between the anterolateral and anterior portals visualization as well as addressing this labral tear with débridement was accomplished successfully, débriding the labrum back to a stable rim. Remaining labrum was then probed and noted to be stable. The débridement was carried down onto the bone just on the undersurface of the labrum without injuring articular cartilage to allow for healing. Final arthroscopic images were obtained. After removal of these cannulas, traction was let down and portal sites were closed with 3-0 Vicryl subcutaneous sutures followed by Steri-Strips. Sterile dressing was applied. The patient was extubated in the operating room and transported to the recovery room without complication. All needle, sponge, and instrument counts were correct.

Answer Sheet

Directions: Be sure to enter all medical record codes in the manner provided in the sample below, paying special attention to the decimal placement for each code. The codes must be typed on the answer sheet in the boxes provided on the computer screen using the keyboard. A decimal point (.) has been provided as a guide for entering each ICD-9-CM code. **You will lose credit if the digits of the codes are correct, but the decimal point has been incorrectly placed.**

CASE 6 DIAGNOSES   **ICD-9-CM**

DX1				.		
DX2				.		
DX3				.		
DX4				.		

CASE 6 PROCEDURES   **CPT/HCPCS**

PR1					
PR2					
PR3					
PR4					
PR5					
PR6					

Practice Cases CASE 7

MR #: 353901

ENDOSCOPY REPORT

PREOPERATIVE DIAGNOSIS: Generalized abdominal pain

POSTOPERATIVE DIAGNOSIS: Grossly normal colonoscopy

RELEVANT HISTORY AND PHYSICAL FINDINGS:

Abdominal pain for years, much improved recently on Activia

MEDICATIONS: None

DIET MODIFICATIONS: Daily Activia

The procedures were explained to the patient including the purpose, the risks, benefits, and possible alternatives procedures were discussed. Consent was obtained. The planned procedures were confirmed with staff and the patient identity was confirmed.

The patient was placed under general anesthesia with ET by anesthesiologist. Photos were taken throughout the procedure. The PCF 160AL was passed via anus. The anus was normally placed. No fissures were observed. No fistulas were observed. No skin tags, no hemorrhoids or rash. The scope was passed. The preparation of the colon at this point was good. The anatomy of the rectum was normal. The mucosa was normal in color and vascularity. Biopsies were taken. The sigmoid anatomy was normal. The mucosa was normal in color and vascularity. Biopsies were taken. Transcending and ascending were both normal appearing. Biopsies taken in the transverse. The cecum was normal. The ICV was visualized and was normal. The terminal ileum was entered. It appeared normal.

COMPLICATIONS: None

The patient was repositioned. The GIF 140 was placed in the mouth and advanced through the mouth and hypopharynx under direct vision. The hypopharynx and cords were normal. Mucosa in the body of the esophagus was normal. The diaphragmatic indentation was visible. The Z line was identified. Biopsies were taken.

The scope was advanced into the stomach which was insufflated with air. The anatomy was normal. Mucosa of the body, antrum, and pylorus were normal. Biopsies were taken of the antrum and body. A turnaround procedure was performed. The gastroesophageal junction was normal. Biopsies were taken in the cardia.

The endoscope was advanced to the third portion of the duodenum. The ampulla of vater was observed. The duodenal folds were normal. The muscosa was normal and velvety. Biopsies ×4 were taken in standard fashion with minimal traction of the duodenal mucosa away from the muscular wall. The jejunum was normal. The endoscope was withdrawn into the stomach which was evacuated of air. The endoscope was removed.

COMPLICATIONS: None

RESULTS: Grossly normal colonoscopy and upper endoscopy

DISPOSITION: The patient was informed of the gross results of the exam. Biopsy results will be reported when received.

Answer Sheet

Directions: Be sure to enter all medical record codes in the manner provided in the sample below, paying special attention to the decimal placement for each code. The codes must be typed on the answer sheet in the boxes provided on the computer screen using the keyboard. A decimal point (.) has been provided as a guide for entering each ICD-9-CM code. **You will lose credit if the digits of the codes are correct, but the decimal point has been incorrectly placed.**

CASE 7 DIAGNOSES   **ICD-9-CM**

				.		
DX1				.		
DX2				.		
DX3				.		
DX4				.		

CASE 7 PROCEDURES   **CPT/HCPCS**

PR1					
PR2					
PR3					
PR4					
PR5					
PR6					

Practice Cases CASE 8

MR #: 641652

DATE: 11-5-20XX

OUTPATIENT INFUSION CLINIC

The patient is a 56-year-old female with iron deficiency anemia with chronic renal failure, stage III moderate, who is here for another dose of iron. She has been doing somewhat better. Her wound is healing up.

She has had blood transfusion of 3 units within the past year. She also has hypertension and type II diabetes.

PLAN: She will be given 1,000 mg of iron today to replenish the lost storage pool. She will resume Aranesp injections at 60 mgs next week. She will see me in the office in 6 weeks.

VITAL SIGNS: 252 lbs, 78 BPM, 140/82, 97.6 oral

MEDICATIONS ORDERED:

Benadryl 50 mg IV push

Infed 1,000 mg IV on 11-5-20XX, start time 9:12 am, end time 12:18 pm

Answer Sheet

Directions: Be sure to enter all medical record codes in the manner provided in the sample below, paying special attention to the decimal placement for each code. The codes must be typed on the answer sheet in the boxes provided on the computer screen using the keyboard. A decimal point (.) has been provided as a guide for entering each ICD-9-CM code. **You will lose credit if the digits of the codes are correct, but the decimal point has been incorrectly placed.**

CASE 8 DIAGNOSES   **ICD-9-CM**

DX1				.	
DX2				.	
DX3				.	
DX4				.	

CASE 8 PROCEDURES   **CPT/HCPCS**

PR1					
PR2					
PR3					
PR4					
PR5					
PR6					

Practice Exam 1
Multiple Choice Questions

Domain 1: Health Information Documentation

1. The physician removes, in his office, a skin lesion from the patient's cheek and submits it to a pathologist for review. The physician documents "skin lesion" in the chart but prior to billing the pathologist reports that it is a basal cell carcinoma. What does the coder submit on the claim form?

   a. Basal cell carcinoma of the skin

   b. Skin lesion

   c. Benign skin lesion

   d. The coder must query the physician because of conflicting data

2. What information is necessary to assign the correct Evaluation and Management (E/M) code for preventive medicine services?

   a. The level of history and examination performed

   b. The counseling provided

   c. The risk factor reduction intervention

   d. The age of the patient

3. What is the best source of documentation to determine the size of a removed malignant lesion?

   a. Pathology report

   b. Postacute care unit record

   c. Operative report

   d. Physical examination

4. A coder might find which of the following on a patient's problem list if the medication list contains the drug Protonix?

   a. High blood pressure

   b. Esophagitis

   c. Congestive heart failure

   d. AIDS

5. The coder notes that the patient is taking prescribed Haldol. The final diagnoses on the progress notes include diabetes mellitus, acute pharyngitis, and malnutrition. What condition might the coder suspect the patient has and should query the physician?

   a. Insomnia

   b. Hypertension

   c. Schizophrenia

   d. Rheumatoid arthritis

6. The patient is seen by the physician and noted to have a chief complaint of shortness of breath. In the progress notes, the physician diagnoses asthma and recommends that the patient present to the Emergency Department of XYZ Hospital immediately. The physician further documents that the patient has severe wheezing and no obvious relief with bronchodilators. What should the coder do when preparing the bill?

   a. Code asthma

   b. Code asthma with status asthmaticus

   c. Code asthma with acute exacerbation

   d. Query the physician for more detail about the asthma

7. A biopsy revealed serous papillary adenocarcinoma. The coder would expect to see a diagnosis of cancer of the:

   a. Bladder

   b. Breast

   c. Ovary

   d. Uterus

8. The coder notes that the physician has ordered potassium replacement for the patient. The coder might expect to see a diagnosis of:

   a. Hypokalemia

   b. Hyponatremia

   c. Hyperkalemia

   d. Hypernatremia

9. Where might a coder find information on whether a particular medication has been administered to the patient?

   a. Physician's orders

   b. Nurse's notes

   c. Problem list

   d. Medical history

Domain 2: ICD-9-CM Diagnosis Coding

10. The physician orders a chest x-ray for a patient who presents with fever, productive cough, and shortness of breath. The physician indicates in the progress notes: Rule out pneumonia. What code(s) should the coder report for the visit when the results have not yet been received?

    a. Pneumonia

    b. Fever, cough, shortness of breath

    c. Cough, shortness of breath

    d. Pneumonia, cough, shortness of breath

11. A series of terms in parentheses sometimes directly following a main term or subterm in ICD-9-CM refers to:

    a. Carryover lines

    b. Exclusion notes

    c. Nonessential modifiers

    d. Eponyms

12. This symbol precedes codes in ICD-9-CM's Tabular Lists of both procedures and diseases and indicates the presence of a footnote at the bottom of the page or references an instructional note located earlier in the section:

    a. Brace

    b. Section mark

    c. Colon

    d. Lozenge

13. This symbol is only found in the Alphabetic Index in ICD-9-CM and encloses a code number that must be used in conjunction with a code immediately preceding it:

    a. Slanted brackets

    b. Parentheses

    c. Square brackets

    d. Brace

14. The coding guideline for late effects is:

    a. Only the residual condition or nature of the late effect is coded

    b. The cause of the late effect is sequenced first followed by the residual condition

    c. Only the cause of the late effect is coded

    d. The residual condition is sequenced first, followed by the cause of the late effect

15. Which of the following would be classified to an ICD-9-CM category for bacterial diseases?

    a. Herpes simplex

    b. *Staphylococcus aureus*

    c. Influenza, types A and B

    d. *Candida albicans*

16. According to ICD-9-CM, an elderly primigravida is defined as a woman who gives birth to her first child after the age of:

    a. 30

    b. 35

    c. 38

    d. 40

17. The physician sees a patient in the hospital because an attempted therapeutic abortion resulted in a liveborn infant. In ICD-9-CM, how would the services provided to the mother be coded?

    a. Use the code for a therapeutic or legal abortion, 635.92

    b. Use the code for the specific type of abortion along with the V30 code (single liveborn)

    c. Use the code for an illegal abortion (636.92) followed by code V27 (outcome of delivery)

    d. Use code 644.21 (early onset of delivery) followed by the outcome of delivery code (V27)

18. Code 650, normal delivery, is assigned for which of the following scenarios:

    a. Delivery resulting in a stillborn

    b. Delivery without prenatal or postpartum complications

    c. Delivery, full-term—breech presentation

    d. Delivery, premature infant with cephalic presentation

19. ICD-9-CM defines the "newborn period" as birth through the _____ day following birth.

    a. 28th

    b. 14th

    c. 60th

    d. 30th

20. "Late pregnancy" (category code 645) is used to demonstrate that a woman is over
    _____ weeks of gestation.

    a. 41

    b. 39

    c. 40

    d. 42

21. In ICD-9-CM, an abnormal communication or opening in the ventricular septum that
    allows blood to shunt from the left ventricle to the right ventricle defines a condition
    known as:

    a. Patent ductus arteriosus

    b. Atrial septal defect

    c. Hypoplastic left ventricle syndrome

    d. Ventricular septal defect

22. How would the following be coded? Physician's office visit: Diagnosis of hypoglycemia
    in infant born to a diabetic mother.

    a. 775.1: Neonatal diabetes mellitus

    b. 250.80: Diabetic hypoglycemia

    c. 775.0: Syndrome of "infant of a diabetic mother"

    d. 250.90: Diabetes with unspecified complication

23. Routine prenatal care, primigravida with no complications would be coded as:

    a. V22.2: Pregnant state, incidental

    b. V22.0: Supervision of normal first pregnancy

    c. V23.9: Unspecified high-risk pregnancy

    d. V22.1: Supervision of other normal pregnancy

24. A woman delivers three babies spontaneously and all babies were liveborn. This would
    be coded as:

651.01 Multiple gestation, twin pregnancy, delivered with or without mention of antepartum condition
651.11 Multiple gestation, triplet pregnancy, delivered with or without mention of antepartum condition
651.91 Multiple gestation, unspecified multiple gestation
V27.5 Outcome of delivery, other multiple birth, all liveborn
V27.6 Outcome of delivery, other multiple birth, some liveborn
V27.9 Outcome of delivery, unspecified outcome of delivery

    a. 651.91; V27.9

    b. 651.11; V27.5

    c. 651.01; V27.6

    d. 651.11; V27.9

Domain 3: CPT and HCPCS II Coding

25. According to the CPT Guidelines, when is it appropriate to code an evaluation and management (E/M) visit based on time?

    a. When the evaluation and management elements for the minimal level have not been met

    b. When counseling and/or coordination of care are more than 50 percent of the visit

    c. When the time spent with the patient exceeds the time listed as typically spent with the patient for that code

    d. When the medical decision making is high and the history and examination are not well-documented

26. The patient presents for an initial insertion of a dual chamber pacemaker. How is this procedure coded?

33206	Insertion or replacement of permanent pacemaker with transvenous electrode(s); atrial
33208	Atrial and ventricular
33216	Insertion of a single transvenous electrode; permanent pacemaker or cardioverter-defibrillator
33217	Insertion of 2 transvenous electrodes, permanent pacemaker or cardioverter-defibrillator

    a. 33206

    b. 33206, 33216

    c. 33208

    d. 33208, 33217

27. A costovertebral approach is used for a posterolateral decompression of the spinal cord. The chest surgeon opens and closes the operative site and the neurosurgeon completes the decompression procedure. Which modifier is applied to the chest surgeon's services?

    a. −54: Surgical care only

    b. −62: Two surgeons

    c. −66: Surgical team

    d. −80: Assistant surgeon

28. When the CPT Index and Tabular Index do not contain a code that describes an adequately documented procedure that was performed by the physician, what action should the coder take?

    a. Assign the code that most closely describes the procedure performed by the physician

    b. Query the physician to determine what the code assignment should be

    c. Assign the unlisted code from the corresponding anatomical section

    d. Assign the code that describes a more complex procedure and attach a −52 modifier

29. The physician completes a percutaneous transluminal coronary angioplasty on a patient with 90 percent blockage of one vessel. How is this service coded?

    a. 92980: Transcatheter placement of an intracoronary stent(s), percutaneous, with or without other therapeutic intervention, any method; single vessel

    b. 92982: Percutaneous transluminal coronary balloon angioplasty; single vessel

    c. 92995: Percutaneous transluminal coronary atherectomy, by mechanical or other method, with or without balloon angioplasty; single vessel

    d. 92997: Percutaneous transluminal pulmonary artery balloon angioplasty; single vessel

30. When coding an E/M code, what modifier would be acceptable for use?

    a. –LT: Left side

    b. –32: Mandated services

    c. –51: Multiple procedures

    d. –59: Distinct procedural service

31. The patient undergoes a TRAM flap reconstruction of the breast. How is this service coded?

    a. 19361: Breast reconstruction with latissimus dorsi flap, without prosthetic implant

    b. 19364: Breast reconstruction with free flap

    c. 19366: Breast reconstruction with other technique

    d. 19367: Breast reconstruction with transverse rectus abdominis myocutaneous flap, single pedicle, including closure of donor site

32. The patient is taken to the operating room by the neurosurgeon for repair of a depressed skull fracture following a motorcycle accident where he was an unhelmeted driver. Two large fragments of skull, one 7 cm and one 6 cm, have pierced the dura. The fragments are removed from the brain along with road contaminate and the dura is repaired. How are the services of the neurosurgeon coded?

    a. 62000: Elevation of depressed skull fracture; simple, extradural

    b. 62005: Elevation of depressed skull fracture; compound or comminuted, extradural

    c. 62010: Elevation of depressed skull fracture; with repair of dura and/or débridement of brain

    d. 62141: Cranioplasty for skull defect; larger than 5 cm in diameter

33. The coder is coding an arthrodesis of the intercarpal joint and the CPT Index has an entry that reads: Arthrodesis, Interphalangeal Joint . . . 26860–26863. What action should the coder take?

    a. Code the first listed code in the series

    b. Code the last listed code in the series

    c. Look up codes 26860 through 26863 and code all the codes

    d. Look up codes 26860 through 26863 and pick the best code

34. When a patient is seen in the office and then admitted as an inpatient and discharged from the hospital all on the same calendar date, what series of codes should the coder use to code these services?

    a. Office and Other Outpatient Services and Hospital Discharge Services

    b. Observation or Inpatient Care Services (including Admission and Discharge Services)

    c. Office and Other Outpatient Services, Initial Hospital Care, and Hospital Discharge Services

    d. Initial Hospital Care and Hospital Discharge Services

35. The patient undergoes a secondary procedure to relieve pressure in the eye. The physician excises a portion of the trabecular meshwork to relieve the pressure. How is this service coded?

    a. 65850: Trabeculotomy ab externo

    b. 65855: Trabeculoplasty by laser surgery, one or more sessions (defined treatment series)

    c. 66170: Fistulization of sclera for glaucoma; trabeculectomy ab externo in absence of previous surgery

    d. 66172: Fistulization of sclera for glaucoma; trabeculectomy ab externo with scarring from previous ocular surgery or trauma

36. The patient lives in an assisted living facility that does not have nursing care. The caregiver calls the patient's physician to see the patient due to severe combativeness during meals. The physician provides an expanded problem-focused history and examination and uses moderate level medical decision making. What code would the physician use to describe these services?

    a. 99213: Office and other outpatient visit for an established patient with expanded problem-focused history and examination and low medical decision making

    b. 99308: Subsequent nursing facility care, per day, with expanded problem-focused history and examination and low medical decision making

    c. 99335: Domiciliary or rest home visit for an established patient with expanded problem-focused history and examination and low medical decision making

    d. 99348: Home visit for an established patient with expanded problem-focused history and examination and low medical decision making

37. A patient with severe cardiac disease undergoes a cardiectomy and transplantation of a replacement heart system. How is this service coded?

    a. 33935: Heart-lung transplant with recipient cardiectomy-pneumonectomy

    b. 33945: Heart transplant, with or without recipient cardiectomy

    c. 0051T: Implantation of a total replacement heart system (artificial heart) with recipient cardiectomy

    d. 0052T: Replacement or repair of thoracic unit of a total replacement heart system (artificial heart)

38. A patient steps on a piece of glass, driving it deep into the plantar surface of the foot. What code does the coder assign for the removal of this glass?

    a. 20525: Removal of foreign body in muscle or tendon sheath; deep or complicated

    b. 28190: Removal of foreign body, foot; subcutaneous

    c. 28192: Removal of foreign body, foot; deep

    d. 28193: Removal of foreign body, foot; complicated

Domain 4: Reimbursement

39. With some insurance plans, the patient pays a fixed amount each time that healthcare services are provided. This fixed amount is called a:

    a. Copayment

    b. Coinsurance

    c. Deductible

    d. Premium

40. The transmission of claims data to payers or clearinghouses is called:

    a. Claims submission

    b. Claims adjudication

    c. Claims arbitration

    d. Claims processing

41. Which of the following is currently used by physicians to submit claims for services provided to patients?

    a. CMS-1500

    b. UB-92

    c. HCFA 1500

    d. UB-04

42. A physician who agrees to accept payment in full of the allowed or approved amount from the Medicare Fee Schedule is called a:

    a. Nonparticipating provider (non-PAR)

    b. Contracted provider

    c. Participating provider (PAR)

    d. Primary provider

43. The total amount of covered medical services that a policyholder must pay for each year before the insurance company will begin to pay is called:

    a. Premium

    b. Coinsurance

    c. Copayment

    d. Deductible

44. Work, practice expense, and malpractice are variables in which government-sponsored reimbursement system?

    a. Resource Based Relative Value Scale (RBRVS) system

    b. Medicare Severity Diagnosis-Related Groups (MS-DRGs)

    c. Ambulatory Payment Classification (APCs)

    d. Resource Utilization Groups (RUGs)

45. What is the name of a waiver required by Medicare for all physician office procedures/services when there is a question as to whether or not the service will be paid for by Medicare?

    a. Assignment of Insurance Benefits

    b. Advance Beneficiary Notice

    c. Explanation of Benefits

    d. Waiver of Medicare Rights

46. What instrument is used to notify the provider with information about payments, denials, and pending status of claims?

    a. Explanation of Benefits

    b. Claims Attachment

    c. Remittance Advice

    d. Medicare Summary Notice

47. How often must an Advance Beneficiary Notice be signed when multiple instances of the same questionable service is provided?

    a. On an annual basis

    b. The first time the questionable service is provided

    c. On a monthly basis

    d. At the time each questionable service is provided

48. What is the purpose of "linking" on a physician claim?

    a. To show how many times a service was provided

    b. To explain medical necessity of a procedure

    c. To group related surgical procedures together

    d. To show the day a procedure was performed

49. The specific legislation that stipulates that ICD-9-CM diagnosis and procedure codes will be issued twice a year, on April 1 and October 1 of each year, is the:

    a. Balanced Budget Act of 1997

    b. Health Information Portability and Accountability Act

    c. Wired for Health Care Quality Act

    d. Medicare Prescription Drug, Improvement, and Modernization Act of 2003

Domain 5: Data Quality and Analysis

50. A coding manager reviewed the following information before the claim was submitted. What change would be required to ensure proper payment?

Patient Name	CPT Code	Description	ICD-9-CM Code	Description
John Doe	30300	Removal of foreign body, intranasal; office type procedure	360.60	Retained foreign body of the eye

   a. A modifier is required on the CPT code.

   b. The diagnosis must be correctly linked to the procedure.

   c. The diagnosis code requires greater specificity.

   d. Additional CPT code(s) are required.

51. Which of the following is the *least* effective way to select an audit sample?

   a. Random sample of records for all physicians in a group

   b. All services provided on a randomly selected day

   c. Records selected by the physician for review

   d. All rejected claims during a specific time period

52. A physician asks how he has been paid for four patients for whom he performed a posterior cervical three-level laminectomy within the past year. Upon review of these claims and the coding, what does the coding manager learn?

63045	Laminectomy, facetectomy and foraminotomy (unilateral or bilateral with decompression of spinal cord, cauda equina and/or nerve root(s), (for example, spinal or lateral recess stenosis), single vertebral segment; cervical
63048	each additional segment, cervical, thoracic, or lumbar (List separately in addition to code for primary procedure.)

	CPT Codes	Diagnosis	Description
Patient 1	63045	722.4	Degeneration of cervical intervertebral disc
Patient 2	63045	722.0	Displacement of cervical intervertebral disc without myelopathy
Patient 3	63045 63048	722.0	Displacement of cervical intervertebral disc without myelopathy
Patient 4	63045 63048	722.4	Degeneration of cervical intervertebral disc

   a. CPT coding accuracy needs improvement.

   b. ICD-9-CM coding accuracy needs improvement.

   c. The physician misidentified patients who received this surgery.

   d. None of the cases was coded correctly.

53. After reviewing this Production Report for June, what action should the coding manager take?

Production Report for Dr. Lyndon, Dermatology 6/1/XX to 6/30/XX				
CPT Code	Frequency	%	Charges	Payments
99212	156	46.2%	$5,772.00	$4,040.40
99213	147	43.6%	$7,350.00	$5,945.00
99214	10	2.9%	$730.00	$511.00
99215	24	7.1%	$2,712.00	$2,316.40
99243	56	65.1 %	$7,000.00	$5,900.00
99244	27	31.3%	$4,050.00	$3,894.00
99245	3	3.4%	$600.00	$492.00

a. Educate Dr. Lyndon about the appropriate use of New Patient codes.

b. Educate Dr. Lyndon on the correct percentages of Consultation codes.

c. Determine why there were so few visits for the month.

d. Investigate why the charges were not paid in full.

Domain 6: Information and Communication Technologies

54. A physician needs a software application that will allow him to computerize his office budget, looking at various categories of expenses such as personnel, office expense, and office supplies and watching patterns of expenditures. What tool would he likely install?

a. Word-processing software

b. Database software

c. Spreadsheet software

d. Database management software

55. The physician is concerned about using the Internet to transmit billing data. The coder assures the physician that the data is protected using:

a. Encryption

b. Encoding

c. Functional interoperability

d. Interface engines

Domain 7: Compliance and Regulatory Issues

56. Which of the following activities would be in violation of AHIMA's Code of Ethics?

    a. Coding an intentionally inappropriate level of service

    b. Following established coding policies and procedures

    c. Protecting the confidentiality of patients' written and electronic records

    d. Taking remedial action when there is direct knowledge of a colleague's incompetence or impairment

57. All of the following organizations make up the Cooperating Parties for the approval of ICD-9-CM coding guidelines **except:**

    a. American Medical Association (AMA)

    b. American Health Information Management Association (AHIMA)

    c. Centers for Medicare and Medicaid Services (CMS)

    d. National Center for Health Statistics (NCHS)

58. One part of a physician's office compliance plan is to respond appropriately to detected violations. Which of the following steps would be a first step of a corrective action plan if the office manager notices that the practice of "unbundling" is commonplace among the coders?

    a. Issue oral warnings to all employees in the department

    b. Refund overpayments from a third-party payer due to this practice

    c. Post the new ICD-9-CM codes each year on the departmental bulletin board

    d. Establish an open-door policy between the physician, the compliance officer, and the employees

59. All of the following are risk areas that the OIG has identified for physician practices **except:**

    a. Billing for noncovered services as if they are covered

    b. Billing for a more expensive service than the one actually performed

    c. Developing, coordinating, and participating in coding training programs

    d. Coding/charging one or two middle levels of service codes exclusively

60. Which of the following is an example of abuse?

    a. Billing for services not provided

    b. Selling or sharing patients' Medicare numbers

    c. Performing services considered by the carrier to be medically unnecessary

    d. Unbundling or exploding charges

Practice Exam 1 Medical Cases

CASE STUDY 1

Please code for the services of the physician.

Practice Exam 1

CASE 1

DATE OF SERVICE: 12/29/20XX

CHIEF COMPLAINT: Flu symptoms, cough

HISTORY OF PRESENT ILLNESS: The patient is an 18-year-old man who is new to my practice and presents to the office today with the following symptoms. Over the past 7 days, he has had diffuse body aches, shortness of breath, cough, productive now, which has changed from initially dry to a greenish-yellow phlegm. He has had some nausea and emesis ×2 today. There has been no diarrhea. He had been taking fluids but decreased appetite. No severe headache, no sore throat, no ear pain. Similar symptoms are in other family members. He presents here with mother for further care and treatment. Approximately 2 days ago, he felt weak and had a brief syncopal episode.

PAST MEDICAL HISTORY: Unremarkable

MEDICATIONS:

1. Wal-Tussin
2. Excedrin

ALLERGIES: SULFA

SOCIAL HISTORY: He smokes continuously approximately two packs per day. Dr. X was his primary care provider in the past. He is here with mother.

REVIEW OF SYSTEMS: See HPI, all other systems reviewed and otherwise negative.

PHYSICAL EXAMINATION:

VITAL SIGNS: Temperature 100.3, blood pressure 130/68, pulse 106, respirations 20, saturation 97% on room air

GENERAL: Awake, alert, nontoxic-appearing male

HEENT: There are well-healed eschars to his right nose and right maxilla region. Pupils are equal and round. Extraocular muscles intact. Tympanic membranes are unremarkable. Mucous membranes are moist. Posterior oropharynx is clear.

NECK: Supple. No rigidity.

CHEST: Some slight crackles in the right base

CARDIOVASCULAR: S1 and S2 normal. Heart tones are crisp. No murmur.

ABDOMEN: Soft, nontender throughout, normoactive bowel tones

EXTREMITIES: Warm, dry, and well perfused. No clubbing, cyanosis, or edema.

NEUROLOGICAL: Nonfocal

His chest x-ray demonstrated an early right middle lobe infiltrate. His white blood cell count was 11.3 with a left shift, 10% bands, 69 segs. His basic chemistry demonstrated a bicarb of 19.2, glucose of 105. The patient was given 500 mg of levaquin IV push under my direct supervision after a sputum and blood cultures ×2. The patient was feeling improved. His temperature did go up to 102 while here, and he was given 1 g of Tylenol orally.

DIAGNOSIS: Right middle lobe pneumonia

DISCHARGE INSTRUCTIONS:

1. Levaquin 500 mg p.o. q.d. a total of 10 days
2. Clear liquids. Advance as tolerated.
3. Phenergan 25 mg per rectum q. 6h. nausea
4. Tylenol 1 g q. 6h. p.r.n.
5. Recommend smoke cessation classes for documented tobacco use disorder

HISTORY: Comprehensive

EXAMINATION: Comprehensive

MEDICAL DECISION MAKING: Moderate

Answer Sheet

Directions: Be sure to enter all medical record codes in the manner provided in the sample below, paying special attention to the decimal placement for each code. The codes must be typed on the answer sheet in the boxes provided on the computer screen using the keyboard. A decimal point (.) has been provided as a guide for entering each ICD-9-CM code. **You will lose credit if the digits of the codes are correct, but the decimal point has been incorrectly placed.**

CASE 1 DIAGNOSES ICD-9-CM

DX1				.		
DX2				.		
DX3				.		
DX4				.		

CASE 1 PROCEDURES CPT/HCPCS

PR1					
PR2					
PR3					
PR4					
PR5					
PR6					

CASE STUDY 2

Please code for the services of the physician.

Practice Exam 1   CASE 2

Inpatient Pulmonary Consultation:

The patient was seen and examined by the intensive care unit house staff. Please see their note for further details. He is posttrauma day 7. Some of his injuries include right acetabulum fracture, right open talus, manubrium rib fracture, mediastinal hematoma, and pulmonary contusion.

This morning, the patient was initially a GCS of 7. We held his sedation. He did wake up and followed some intermittent commands. He is currently on morphine at 2 mg/hour and Ativan at 2 mg/hour.

His lungs are coarse bilaterally. He is on assist control, rate of 12, tidal volume 600, PEEP of 10, FIO_2 of 0.4. His saturations have been greater than 96%. He persists in acute respiratory failure; however, his AA gradient has been improving and we will attempt to decrease his PEEP today. Patient has a pulmonary contusion which I will continue to monitor.

Cardiovascular: His pulse is 80 to 115, blood pressure 100 to 130/60 to 80. He is in sinus tachycardia on examination.

Renal/fluid/electrolytes: He had 3.4 liters in and 2.4 liters out. His glucoses have been well controlled with Endotool. His electrolytes are all within normal limits. His abdomen is much less distended than it has been over the previous several days. He is receiving tube feeds at 65 cc/hour. He has had four bowel movements.

Hematology: His hemoglobin is stable at 10. His platelet count is 225. He has on SCDs and is receiving Lovenox for DVT prophylaxis. T-max is 101.3. There is a much improved temperature curve and his white blood cell count is down to 11 from 12. He is currently on Linezolid and tobramycin. His BAL from 09/09 grew out *Haemophilus influenzae* and now yeast. His urine and blood cultures from 09/12 are negative. We will start Diflucan today. We will also send stool for C-diff. We will await final cultures from BAL prior to discontinuing Linezolid. We will continue tobramycin for treatment of his *Haemophilus influenzae*.

I spent over 30 minutes at this patient's bedside assessing him and making critical care decisions.

Answer Sheet

Directions: Be sure to enter all medical record codes in the manner provided in the sample below, paying special attention to the decimal placement for each code. The codes must be typed on the answer sheet in the boxes provided on the computer screen using the keyboard. A decimal point (.) has been provided as a guide for entering each ICD-9-CM code. **You will lose credit if the digits of the codes are correct, but the decimal point has been incorrectly placed.**

CASE 2 DIAGNOSES   **ICD-9-CM**

DX1				.		
DX2				.		
DX3				.		
DX4				.		

CASE 2 PROCEDURES   **CPT/HCPCS**

PR1					
PR2					
PR3					
PR4					
PR5					
PR6					

CASE STUDY 3

Please code for the services of the physician.

Practice Exam 1

CASE 3

OFFICE VISIT

CHIEF COMPLAINT: Diarrhea and nausea

HISTORY OF PRESENT ILLNESS: This is a 70-year-old Caucasian male, established patient, who presents today to the office with complaints of diarrhea, and nausea present over the last 6 weeks that have increased gradually in frequency. Currently, he's having diarrhea that's three times a day. It's watery at times, sometimes soft. He thinks that things are worsening. The color of the stool is tan or brown. He has no black or tarry stools. He notes no bright red blood per rectum. He does admit to lethargy.

Upon questioning, he does admit to being on an antibiotic recently, approximately 6 weeks ago. Before his symptoms started, he had been put on Z-Pak for some sinus symptoms, and he did notice that his symptoms started after being on the Z-Pak.

He was started on Prilosec several weeks ago for some irritation due to Fosamax and he has been on Prilosec since then.

In addition, he relates today that he was scratched by some dogs and according to our chart, hasn't had a tetanus shot since 1998.

PAST MEDICAL HISTORY:

Numerous medical issues, in particular:

1. Cardiac issues
2. Hypertension
3. Hypercholesterolemia

CURRENT MEDICATIONS:

1. Aspirin
2. Calcium
3. Ticlid
4. Zocor
5. Prilosec

SOCIAL HISTORY: He denies alcohol or tobacco.

REVIEW OF SYSTEMS: Negative for chest pain or shortness of breath. He does admit to increased flatulence and abdominal pain, only after eating, which resolves after the flatulence resolves.

PHYSICAL EXAMINATION:

VITAL SIGNS: BLOOD PRESSURE: 120/54. PULSE: 56. TEMPERATURE: 98.1. WEIGHT: 135

GENERAL: He is in no acute distress. Able to give a good history. He's alert and oriented without evidence of severe lethargy or fatigue.

HEART: Regular rate and rhythm. No murmurs, gallops, or rubs or heaves.

LUNGS: Clear to auscultation

ABDOMEN: Soft and nontender. No organomegaly. Hyperactive bowel sounds. No skin changes.

EXTREMITIES: Without cyanosis, clubbing, or edema

SKIN: No abnormalities, except for several abrasions and excoriations on his anterior arms due to dogs scratching at him today.

ASSESSMENT AND PLAN:

1. I gave him a Td shot today. The abrasions are somewhat deep and have some debris. I cleansed the one on the right forearm and rebandaged it.

2. With regard to his significant diarrhea, I do want to rule out C. differential, so will send off a stool for C. differential blood count toxin. Also will send off a culture to rule out *Salmonella, Shigella,* or entero Campylobacter, and I've also asked him to stop the Prilosec right now to see if his symptoms improve off Prilosec as this may be an offending agent as well.

All questions were answered. He will return the stool sample in the morning.

HISTORY: Detailed

EXAMINATION: Detailed

MEDICAL DECISION MAKING: Moderate

Answer Sheet

Directions: Be sure to enter all medical record codes in the manner provided in the sample below, paying special attention to the decimal placement for each code. The codes must be typed on the answer sheet in the boxes provided on the computer screen using the keyboard. A decimal point (.) has been provided as a guide for entering each ICD-9-CM code. **You will lose credit if the digits of the codes are correct, but the decimal point has been incorrectly placed.**

CASE 3 DIAGNOSES ICD-9-CM

DX1				.		
DX2				.		
DX3				.		
DX4				.		

CASE 3 PROCEDURES CPT/HCPCS

PR1					
PR2					
PR3					
PR4					
PR5					
PR6					

CASE STUDY 4

Please code for the services of the physician.

Practice Exam 1

CASE 4

DATE OF ADMISSION: 01/15/20XX

DATE OF CONSULTATION: 01/15/20XX

REQUESTED BY: Dr. Y

CHIEF COMPLAINT: Not feeling good and constipation

CONSULT SERVICE: Endocrinology (patient to be transferred from unit and will be on the Endocrine Service)

HISTORY OF PRESENT ILLNESS: The patient is a 4-year-old boy who was taken to the emergency department by his parents because he had constipation and he was subsequently admitted as an inpatient. He has had no stools for 5 days. He also began vomiting the morning of admission. He has had decreased food intake over the past 5 days. He has had polyuria and polydipsia for past 2 months, also bedwetting for 1 to 2 months. He has had a 7-lb weight loss. He had not been complaining of abdominal pain, no complaints of blurred vision, no complaints of headache.

In the emergency department, by mom's report, he was given an enema. They also elected to do some labs. He was found to have a blood sugar level over 400 and a pH of 7.10. He was admitted to the pediatric intensive care unit.

PAST MEDICAL HISTORY: He was the product of a normal pregnancy. Birth weight 8 lb 10 oz. He has had no hospitalizations. He has no known drug allergies.

FAMILY HISTORY: Negative for type 1 diabetes. There is type 2 diabetes only in a maternal great-grandmother. There is a maternal grandmother with rheumatoid arthritis, thyroid problems, cardiovascular disease (had CABG in mid-40s) and dyslipidemia. Mom is not aware of any issues regarding health on maternal grandfather's side of the family, but admittedly does not know much about her father's history. His father is Filipino/Samoan ethnicity, knows of no diabetes in the family and no major health problems. The patient has a 2-year-old brother who is healthy. Mom is 35 weeks' pregnant. She has had no gestational diabetes. Father had some cold symptoms, and the patient developed cold symptoms also in the past week.

SOCIAL HISTORY: The patient lives with his parents and sibling.

REVIEW OF SYMPTOMS: Negative for fever or fatigue. There has been a 5- to 7-lb weight loss as mentioned above. Nasal discharge as mentioned above, no complaints of sore throat, mild cough, no chest pain, decreased appetite, vomiting as mentioned above and constipation as mentioned above, polyuria, polydipsia, nocturia, no dysuria, no weakness, no headaches. Regarding mood changes, mom has noted that he has seemed to have more behavioral issues upon eating sugar. Mom does believe his skin and lips to be dry for the past few weeks.

PHYSICAL EXAMINATION: The patient is an alert, smiling boy in no distress. Weight 25.1 kg, temperature 36.7, pulse 119, respiratory rate 18, blood pressure 99/79

> **HEENT:** Conjunctivae normal. Pupils reactive. Glimpses of his fundi normal. Oral mucosa moist. Breath not fruity in odor. No oropharyngeal exudate.

> **NECK:** Supple with no thyroid enlargement

> **LUNGS:** Clear, no wheezing

> **CARDIAC:** Normal rhythm, no murmur

> **ABDOMEN:** Soft, nontender, normal bowel sounds

> **GENITALIA:** He had normal prepubertal genitalia. Testes descended bilaterally.

> **SKIN:** Notable for 2 small café-au-lait spots on his trunk, slightly doughy texture of his skin

> **NEUROLOGIC:** Sensation was grossly intact. He had normal speech.

LABORATORY STUDIES: On admission, venous pH 7.10, blood glucose 449, sodium 144, potassium 4.3, chloride 110, CO_2 less than 5, BUN 7, creatinine 0.6. calcium 11.2, magnesium 2.2, phosphorus 4.2. CBC was remarkable for a white blood cell count of 13.5, 63 polys, 22 lymphocytes, 10 monocytes, hematocrit 46.3. Hemoglobin A1c pending at the time of this dictation.

IMPRESSION: This is a 4-year-old with new-onset diabetes, presenting in severe diabetic ketoacidosis (DKA). His DKA is resolving. DKA management as per diabetes clinical pathway, he is currently on an insulin infusion at 0.1 units per kg/hour and D10 fluids. Blood glucose checked q2h, electrolytes q4h at present. He will be transitioned to subcutaneous insulin later in the day, starting at 1 unit per kg per day. In view of the family situation, with mom's upcoming delivery, likely NPH and Humalog insulin will be a bit easier for this family. Diabetes education will begin today with diabetes nurse educator, later in the week nutritionist and social worker.

Regarding constipation, we will continue to follow this. Also, of note is the fact that on his initial studies he had 2+ protein as well as ketonuria. Would recheck urinalysis later during his hospital stay.

HISTORY: Comprehensive

EXAMINATION: Comprehensive

MEDICAL DECISION MAKING: High

Answer Sheet

Directions: Be sure to enter all medical record codes in the manner provided in the sample below, paying special attention to the decimal placement for each code. The codes must be typed on the answer sheet in the boxes provided on the computer screen using the keyboard. A decimal point (.) has been provided as a guide for entering each ICD-9-CM code. **You will lose credit if the digits of the codes are correct, but the decimal point has been incorrectly placed.**

CASE 4 DIAGNOSES   **ICD-9-CM**

DX1				.		
DX2				.		
DX3				.		
DX4				.		

CASE 4 PROCEDURES   **CPT/HCPCS**

PR1					
PR2					
PR3					
PR4					
PR5					
PR6					

CASE STUDY 5

Please code for the services of the physician.

Practice Exam 1

CASE 5

CHIEF COMPLAINT: Persistent vaginal bleeding, follow-up to spontaneous AB

HISTORY OF PRESENT ILLNESS: The patient is a 30-year-old woman who presents to the emergency room with the chief complaint of persistent vaginal bleeding and cramping. The patient was seen here on January 22. At that time, she reported being 8 weeks pregnant. She had a complete evaluation that included a beta hCG of 514, an ultrasound that showed no contents within the uterus. She was thought to have had a completed spontaneous AB. She states that she has had persistent cramping and bleeding and also is interested in the results of her follow-up beta hCG. This is the patient's second pregnancy. She has had a previous spontaneous AB. Past medical history is also significant for anxiety, depression, and anemia.

CURRENT MEDICATIONS:

1. Clonazepam
2. Trazodone
3. Amitriptyline
4. Vitamin B_{12}

She is taking nothing until she knows for sure whether or not she is pregnant.

ALLERGIES: She states she is allergic to SULFA.

SOCIAL HISTORY: She is an occasional smoker.

FAMILY HISTORY: Noncontributory

REVIEW OF SYSTEMS: There is no history of headache, nosebleed, syncope, seizure, cough or cold symptoms, vomiting, diarrhea, other joint aches or pains, or rash.

PHYSICAL EXAMINATION:

VITAL SIGNS: Blood pressure 104/79, pulse rate 81, respiratory rate 16, temperature 96.8. O_2 sat remains at 100%.

GENERAL: The patient is awake, alert, somewhat flat affect, no acute distress.

> **HEENT:** Skull is atraumatic. Pupils are reactive. Fundi are normal. TMs are clear. There were no oral lesions.
>
> **NECK:** Supple without adenopathy
>
> **LUNGS:** Clear
>
> **HEART:** Tones are normal
>
> **ABDOMEN:** Soft. Completely nontender.
>
> **PELVIC:** Examination performed by me showed normal genitalia, normal mucosa, a nulliparous os. The os was closed. Uterine size was consistent with a nonpregnant uterus. There was no bleeding present at all and no adnexal tenderness.

EXTREMITIES: No cyanosis, clubbing, or edema

NEUROLOGICAL: The patient is intact.

The patient was thought to have a completed spontaneous AB. Hemoglobin and hematocrit are 13 and 39 demonstrating no evidence of anemia. Beta hCG that was 514 on January 22 is now 35. Urinalysis did reveal a UTI. Patient was started on Urimar. She was assured that she has had a completed AB and should expect light bleeding and cramping over the next week and will follow up for any further complications. She was sent home in stable condition.

DIAGNOSIS: Prior spontaneous AB, complete; UTI

HISTORY: Detailed

EXAMINATION: Comprehensive

MEDICAL DECISION-MAKING: Moderate

Answer Sheet

Directions: Be sure to enter all medical record codes in the manner provided in the sample below, paying special attention to the decimal placement for each code. The codes must be typed on the answer sheet in the boxes provided on the computer screen using the keyboard. A decimal point (.) has been provided as a guide for entering each ICD-9-CM code. **You will lose credit if the digits of the codes are correct, but the decimal point has been incorrectly placed.**

CASE 5 DIAGNOSES   **ICD-9-CM**

DX1				.		
DX2				.		
DX3				.		
DX4				.		

CASE 5 PROCEDURES   **CPT/HCPCS**

PR1					
PR2					
PR3					
PR4					
PR5					
PR6					

CASE STUDY 6

Please code for the services of the physician and the office.

Practice Exam 1   CASE 6

Dr. Y
Northwest Health Center

Dear Dr. Y:

We had the pleasure of seeing your patient at the Cardiology Clinic today, March 2, 20XX. As you know, he is a 10-year-old boy, who was sent for evaluation of an irregular heartbeat. He had an electrocardiogram performed on January 31, 20XX after detection of an irregular heart rate on physical examination. This study demonstrated ventricular bigeminy, and the coupling interval at that time on the PVCs was approximately 500 milliseconds. Patient has had no symptoms referable to the cardiac system. Specifically, he denies any history of exercise intolerance, chest pain, palpitations, syncope or presyncope, or cyanosis. Other than occasional headaches, he has no significant past medical history. His family history is negative for cardiac disease in children. He takes no medications, has no known medication allergies, and his immunizations are up to date by report.

On physical examination today, his height was 141.8 cm, his weight was 35.9 kg, his heart rate was 90, his respiratory rate was 21, and his blood pressure in the right upper extremity was 114/51 and in the left upper extremity, it was 101/54. In the right lower extremity, it was 107/52 and in the left lower extremity, it was 105/67. In general, he is well developed and well nourished, in no apparent distress. He is normocephalic and nondysmorphic, with moist mucous membranes and no central cyanosis. He has a large café-au-lait spot on the abdomen. The chest is symmetrical and clear to auscultation bilaterally. The cardiac examination demonstrates a quiet precordium, with no heave or thrill. The rate was regular with normal S1, and physiologic splitting of S2. There are no murmurs, clicks, gallops or rubs appreciated. The abdomen was soft and nontender with no hepatosplenomegaly. The extremities are warm and well perfused with 2+ pulses distally, no brachiofemoral delay, and no cyanosis, clubbing, or edema.

An echocardiogram was performed today that demonstrated normal anatomy and function.

It is our impression that he is doing very well from a cardiac standpoint. He appears to be in a persistent bigeminy pattern, with preserved cardiac function. In the absence of structural heart disease, which is ruled out by the echocardiogram, this abnormal rhythm should resolve spontaneously in time. We would like to see him again in the cardiology clinic for follow-up with a repeat electrocardiogram in 1 year. In the meantime, he will not require SBE prophylaxis or exercise restriction.

Thank you for allowing us to participate in the care of this patient. Please do not hesitate to contact us with questions or concerns.

Very truly yours,

Dr. Z

cc Dr. W

HISTORY: Expanded Problem Focused

EXAMINATION: Detailed

MEDICAL DECISION-MAKING: Low

PEDIATRIC ECHOCARDIOGRAPHY REPORT

Requested by: Dr. Y

Sonographer: Dr. W

Reason for test: Irregular beats

Procedures: 2-D ECHO, Doppler, Doppler Color Flow

Measure

Function

	Value	Unit	Z Score	Min	Max
LV diastolic dimension	3.43	cm	−2.38	3.55	4.90
LV systolic dimension	1.91	cm	−3.45	2.23	3.35
LV shortening fraction	44.31	%			
LV diastolic wall thickness	0.61	cm	−1.69	0.59	0.98
Diastolic septal thickness	0.62	cm	−1.48	0.57	1.08
M-mode LV mass	51.71	gm	−3.13	65.26	143.65

A-V Canal

Tricuspid regurgitation, trivial

Conotruncus

Pulmonary regurgitation, trivial

Great Arteries

Normal coronary artery origins and courses

Other

Left aortic arch with normal branching

No structural defects identified

Report Comment: Normal anatomy and function

Answer Sheet

Directions: Be sure to enter all medical record codes in the manner provided in the sample below, paying special attention to the decimal placement for each code. The codes must be typed on the answer sheet in the boxes provided on the computer screen using the keyboard. A decimal point (.) has been provided as a guide for entering each ICD-9-CM code. **You will lose credit if the digits of the codes are correct, but the decimal point has been incorrectly placed.**

CASE 6 DIAGNOSES — ICD-9-CM

DX1				.		
DX2				.		
DX3				.		
DX4				.		

CASE 6 PROCEDURES — CPT/HCPCS

PR1					
PR2					
PR3					
PR4					
PR5					
PR6					

CASE STUDY 7

Please code for the services of the surgeon.

Practice Exam 1 **CASE 7**

DATE OF BIRTH: 08/30/1949

ADMISSION DATE: 12/13/20XX

SURGERY DATE: 12/13/20XX

PREOPERATIVE DIAGNOSIS: Thyroid nodule

POSTOPERATIVE DIAGNOSIS: Necrotic thyroid nodule, Hashimoto's thyroiditis based on frozen section.

PROCEDURE: Right thyroid lobectomy and frozen section

ESTIMATED BLOOD LOSS: 30 mL

With adequate sedation in the operating room, the patient was given a general anesthetic. The patient was positioned and prepared and draped for thyroidectomy. A collar incision was performed after the skin was appropriately marked for symmetry. The skin, subcutaneous tissue, and platysmal muscle were divided, and then superior-inferior flaps were developed behind the platysmal muscle. The strap muscles were separated in the midline. There was a dominant nodule in the right lobe of the thyroid. The left lobe appeared grossly normal, although slightly enlarged and fleshy. Previous imaging had demonstrated some cystic change in the left lobe as well, but this was not apparent on gross examination. The right thyroid lobe was mobilized first by double ligating the superior thyroid vessels and then transected, and the thyroid gland mobilized. The parathyroid glands were not definitely visualized, but care was taken to dissect exactly on the capsule of the thyroid lobe. The recurrent laryngeal nerve was carefully identified and preserved. The inferior thyroidal vessels were clamped, transected, and ligated. Other bleeders were identified and secured with ligatures of 3-0 silk as well. The isthmus was transected and transfixed with two transfixion stitches of 3-0 silk. Hemostasis was then satisfactory. Frozen section revealed a mass with a necrotic center and a thin wall, which showed no malignant change. Permanent sections pending. The strap muscles were then approximated in the midline with a running simple stitch of 3-0 Vicryl. The platysmal muscle was approximated with interrupted simple stitches of 3-0 Vicryl and the skin was closed with 4-0 Vicryl. A sterile dressing was applied and the patient left the operating room in satisfactory condition having tolerated the procedure satisfactorily.

Answer Sheet

Directions: Be sure to enter all medical record codes in the manner provided in the sample below, paying special attention to the decimal placement for each code. The codes must be typed on the answer sheet in the boxes provided on the computer screen using the keyboard. A decimal point (.) has been provided as a guide for entering each ICD-9-CM code. **You will lose credit if the digits of the codes are correct, but the decimal point has been incorrectly placed.**

CASE 7 DIAGNOSES   **ICD-9-CM**

DX1				.		
DX2				.		
DX3				.		
DX4				.		

CASE 7 PROCEDURES   **CPT/HCPCS**

PR1					
PR2					
PR3					
PR4					
PR5					
PR6					

CASE STUDY 8

Please code for the services of the surgeon.

Practice Exam 1   CASE 8

DATE OF PROCEDURE: 10/30/20XX

PREOPERATIVE DIAGNOSIS: Left quadriceps tendon rupture

POSTOPERATIVE DIAGNOSIS: Left quadriceps tendon rupture

PROCEDURE: Repair of left quadriceps tendon rupture

ANESTHESIA: Spinal

COMPLICATIONS: None

DRAINS: None

ESTIMATED BLOOD LOSS: 50 cc to 100 cc

PROCEDURE: The patient was brought to the operating room and after the instillation of a satisfactory spinal anesthesia, the left lower extremity was appropriately prepared and draped in the usual sterile fashion. A midline incision was made and centered over the patella and carried down to the quadriceps mechanism. Medial and lateral dissection was carried out to expose the retinaculum, which was torn approximately 2 cm laterally and medially. There was a direct avulsion of the quadriceps tendon off the patella with a small fleck of osteophytic bone. The quadriceps tendon was freshened. Also the bony surface of the patella was débrided of soft tissue and hematoma and fibrous tissue. Once this was repaired, three holes, center, mid lateral, and mid medial were marked. Following this, a #5 Ethibond and #2 fiberwire were placed in the quadriceps mechanism both medially and laterally, beginning in the midportion with a Krackow suture. Following this, three drill holes were made longitudinally from superior to inferior through the patella and a suture passer was used to retrieve the ends of the suture. When these were secured, the quad tendon was brought down into the patellar bed. Following this, #2 Ethibond retinacular sutures were added from the superolateral and superomedial junction of the patella laterally and medially. These were then tightened. As they were tightened, the sutures in the patella were securely tightened as well. The retinacular sutures were then tightened. Supplemental 2-0 Vicryl anteriorly into the quad tendon and patellar soft tissue and retinaculum was then accomplished. This knee could be flexed to about 30 degrees before there was significant tension on this quadriceps tendon. Therefore, we will be holding him in extension. Following this, a thorough Water Pik irrigation was accomplished. The subcutaneous was closed with interrupted 2-0 Vicryl and the skin closed with skin clips. A sterile dressing and a knee immobilizer were placed. The patient was taken to the recovery room in satisfactory condition.

Answer Sheet

Directions: Be sure to enter all medical record codes in the manner provided in the sample below, paying special attention to the decimal placement for each code. The codes must be typed on the answer sheet in the boxes provided on the computer screen using the keyboard. A decimal point (.) has been provided as a guide for entering each ICD-9-CM code. **You will lose credit if the digits of the codes are correct, but the decimal point has been incorrectly placed.**

CASE 8 DIAGNOSES   **ICD-9-CM**

				.		
DX1				.		
DX2				.		
DX3				.		
DX4				.		

CASE 8 PROCEDURES   **CPT/HCPCS**

PR1					
PR2					
PR3					
PR4					
PR5					
PR6					

CASE STUDY 9

Please code for the services of the surgeon.

Practice Exam 1   CASE 9

DATE OF PROCEDURE: 09/14/20XX

PREOPERATIVE DIAGNOSIS: Right tibia nonunion with open lateral wound

POSTOPERATIVE DIAGNOSIS: Right tibia nonunion with open lateral wound

PROCEDURES PERFORMED: Split-thickness skin graft to right lower extremity for wound coverage

ANESTHESIA: General endotracheal anesthesia

BLOOD LOSS: None

FLUIDS: 1,400 cc of LR

INDICATIONS FOR THE PROCEDURE: The patient had poor healing of a wound status post right tibial nonunion of an open fracture. Patient was involved in auto accident 6 months ago. Risks, benefits, and alternatives of the procedure were explained to the patient in full detail. The patient is in agreement with the plan and is agreeable to proceeding with the operation.

PROCEDURE: The patient was brought to the operating suite and placed supine on the operating room table. Following administration of general endotracheal anesthesia, the right lower extremity was prepared and draped in sterile fashion. The entire right leg was prepared with antiseptic solution and adequately draped in a sterile manner.

Attention was first directed to the lateral right lower extremity wound and the most proximal edges were débrided back to bleeding edges with a small curette to remove devitalized, necrotic skin. The rest of the wound was deemed to look healthy with viable skin edges and excellent granulation tissue. Attention was then turned to the donor site on the ipsilateral leg using a dermatome at 12 one thousandths of an inch. A skin graft from the right thigh was taken and meshed on a template. The meshed skin graft was then placed over the lateral lower extremity wound. The skin graft covered an area of 85 sq cm. The skin graft adequately covered the wound. The edges of the skin graft were contoured to approximate the edges of the wound. Staples were used to fix the skin graft. Xeroform was then used to cover both the donor and recipient site and Owens gauze was applied on top of the piriform. The wounds were then dressed with ABDs, cotton wrapping, and bias. The patient was then awakened and returned to the recovery room in good condition.

Answer Sheet

Directions: Be sure to enter all medical record codes in the manner provided in the sample below, paying special attention to the decimal placement for each code. The codes must be typed on the answer sheet in the boxes provided on the computer screen using the keyboard. A decimal point (.) has been provided as a guide for entering each ICD-9-CM code. **You will lose credit if the digits of the codes are correct, but the decimal point has been incorrectly placed.**

CASE 9 DIAGNOSES   **ICD-9-CM**

DX1				.		
DX2				.		
DX3				.		
DX4				.		

CASE 9 PROCEDURES   **CPT/HCPCS**

PR1					
PR2					
PR3					
PR4					
PR5					
PR6					

CASE STUDY 10

Please code for the services of the surgeon.

Practice Exam 1   CASE 10

DATE OF OPERATION: 01/30/20XX

PREOPERATIVE DIAGNOSIS: Multiple myeloma with pending stem cell transplant

POSTOPERATIVE DIAGNOSIS: Multiple myeloma with pending stem cell transplant

PROCEDURE: Placement of tunneled central venous Neostar catheter via the right internal jugular vein with ultrasound and fluoroscopic assistance.

ANESTHESIA: Local with MAC

ESTIMATED BLOOD LOSS: Minimal

FLUIDS: 750 mL of crystalloid

DRAINS: None

SPECIMENS: None

COMPLICATIONS: None

INDICATIONS: This patient is a 47-year-old man with a diagnosis of multiple myeloma. Stem cell transplantation is pending and the patient is in need of a central venous catheter suitable for pheresis.

PROCEDURE: After obtaining informed consent, the patient was brought to the operating room and placed supine on the operating table. The skin of the anterior chest and neck was shaved, prepared, and draped in the standard sterile fashion. Using ultrasound guidance by Dr X, a needle with syringe was advanced into the internal jugular vein with good blood return. A larger introducer needle was then advanced parallel to the previous needle under ultrasound guidance and placed into the right internal jugular vein with good blood return. A guidewire was advanced through the introducer needle under fluoroscopic guidance. The needle was then removed, leaving the guidewire in place. A 5-mm incision was made at the site of the wire exiting the skin with a #11 blade scalpel. It should be noted that the skin of the right neck was anesthetized with 1% lidocaine for analgesia. At this point, a suitable location in the right chest was chosen for the catheter exit site.

This area, as well as the subcutaneous tract, were anesthetized with 1% lidocaine. A 5-mm skin incision was made at the anticipated catheter exit site with a #11 blade scalpel. A tunneler device was then used to create the subcutaneous tunnel, bringing the tunneler in a cephalad fashion and out through the previous skin incision in the neck.

At this point, a dilator was passed over the guidewire under fluoroscopy to dilate the tract. This was done serially. An introducer peel-away catheter was threaded over the guidewire, and the guidewire was then removed. The previously tunneled Neostar catheter was then advanced through the peel-away sheath under fluoroscopy. The sheath was removed, and the catheter had a good position in the cavoatrial junction. There was an acute angle in the catheter site as it exited the fascia of the neck. This was corrected by extending the skin incision and creating a nice curve in the catheter without kinks. Again, distal placement was confirmed at the cavoatrial junction under live fluoroscopy. The catheter withdrew blood and flushed easily at all three ports. One thousand units per cc of heparin flush were used to hep-lock the catheter. The catheter was secured to the skin of the right chest with a 4-0 prolene suture. A 4-0 Vicryl was then used to reapproximate the skin of the neck incision. Derma-bond was applied to the neck incision site, and sterile dressings were applied. The patient tolerated the procedure well and without any complications. A chest x-ray is pending in the recovery room to confirm adequate placement of the catheter and to rule out a pneumothorax.

Answer Sheet

Directions: Be sure to enter all medical record codes in the manner provided in the sample below, paying special attention to the decimal placement for each code. The codes must be typed on the answer sheet in the boxes provided on the computer screen using the keyboard. A decimal point (.) has been provided as a guide for entering each ICD-9-CM code. **You will lose credit if the digits of the codes are correct, but the decimal point has been incorrectly placed.**

CASE 10 DIAGNOSES   **ICD-9-CM**

DX1				.		
DX2				.		
DX3				.		
DX4				.		

CASE 10 PROCEDURES   **CPT/HCPCS**

PR1					
PR2					
PR3					
PR4					
PR5					
PR6					

CASE STUDY 11

Please code for the services of the surgeon.

Practice Exam 1   CASE 11

PREOPERATIVE DIAGNOSIS: End-stage renal disease

POSTOPERATIVE DIAGNOSIS: End-stage renal disease

OPERATION: Left brachiocephalic arteriovenous fistula

ESTIMATED BLOOD LOSS: Less than 25 cc

COMPLICATIONS: None

PROCEDURE: The patient was taken to the operating room and placed in the supine position, where his left arm was placed on an arm board and prepared and draped in the usual sterile fashion. He was given intravenous sedation and a local anesthetic using 1% lidocaine. After infiltration of the area just above the antecubital fossa, an incision was made between the brachial artery and the cephalic vein and approximately 1 cm beyond the antecubital fossa proximally toward the shoulder. This was carried down through the skin and subcutaneous tissues to the level of the fascia. The fascia was identified, and dissection was continued laterally and medially to expose the cephalic vein, which was noted to have a medial branch that was large and clotted and a lateral branch that was a little smaller but clearly open. We traced the cephalic vein distally and proximally and developed enough mobility of the vein with ligation of branches and surrounding tissues to be able to move it toward the brachial artery for close approximation for anastomosis. Attention was then turned to the brachial artery, which was identified in a somewhat deep position in the medial aspect of the elbow and was noted to be relatively small with a diameter of around 4 to 5 mm. It had some mild disease in the arterial wall; however, after ligation of a single small branch, we were able to get elevation of approximately 2.5 cm of the artery. This provided adequate exposure for the arteriotomy and for proximal and distal occlusion. The patient then had amputation and ligation of the cephalic vein distally with the cut end being brought over to the artery. The artery itself was opened with a #11 blade after proximal and distal occlusion, and approximately 6 mm of anastomosis was performed in running fashion with 6-0 prolene using the end of the spatulated cephalic vein to the side of the brachial artery. The patient tolerated this procedure very well. The anastomosis, once completed, did not bleed, and there was a good thrill in the vein. After inspection, there was no evidence of any significant obstruction to the vein course and no kinking that would cause any problems with development of the fistula.

At this point, we infiltrated the wounds with 0.25% Marcaine for postoperative anesthesia and closed the wounds with interrupted 3-0 Vicryl for the subcutaneous tissues and running 4-0 Monocryl for the skin. Sponge and needle counts were correct, and the patient was taken to recovery without incident with plan for discharge.

Answer Sheet

Directions: Be sure to enter all medical record codes in the manner provided in the sample below, paying special attention to the decimal placement for each code. The codes must be typed on the answer sheet in the boxes provided on the computer screen using the keyboard. A decimal point (.) has been provided as a guide for entering each ICD-9-CM code. **You will lose credit if the digits of the codes are correct, but the decimal point has been incorrectly placed.**

CASE 11 DIAGNOSES ICD-9-CM

					.		
DX1					.		
DX2					.		
DX3					.		
DX4					.		

CASE 11 PROCEDURES CPT/HCPCS

PR1					
PR2					
PR3					
PR4					
PR5					
PR6					

CASE STUDY 12

Please code for the services of the surgeon.

Practice Exam 1   CASE 12

DATE OF OPERATION: 01/05/20XX

PREOPERATIVE DIAGNOSIS: Congenital cataract of the right eye

POSTOPERATIVE DIAGNOSIS: Congenital cataract of the right eye

OPERATION: Cataract extraction with primary posterior capsulotomy and limited anterior vitrectomy with intraocular lens.

INDICATIONS: Patient with a congenital cataract of the right eye, needed to have surgical intervention to remove it, which was performed here today.

ANESTHESIA: General orotracheal anesthesia

ESTIMATED BLOOD LOSS: Negligible

COMPLICATIONS: None

SPECIMENS SENT TO PATHOLOGY: None

PROCEDURE IN DETAIL: The patient was brought back to the operating room, adequately premedicated and intubated without complications. Directly after induction, the patient had pressures taken in both eyes and was found to have a pressure in the right eye of 16 and in the left eye of 17.

That was within 2 minutes of induction, error rate less than 5%.

Then keratometry readings were performed, three sets of two readings on each eye. On the right eye 44.5 × 46.25. Second reading is 44 × 46.25. The third reading is 44.5 × 46. In the left eye, 44.75 × 45, 44.25 × 45 and 43.75 × 45. Central corneal thickness for the right eye was 593 microns ± 1.5 microns and left eye 562 microns ± 1.8 microns. Axial lengths were then measured using I^3 ultrasound. For the right eye, the axial length was found to be 20.28 and the left eye 20.44. With the given K's and the axial lengths for the right eye, it was determined that for approximately 2 to 2.5 undercorrection, a 27.5 lens needed to be put in his eye and that was the one that was chosen.

Then the patient was prepared and draped in the usual sterile ophthalmic fashion after he received several mydriatic and cycloplegic drops. He also received one drop of Ciloxan to the right eye every 5 minutes for three drops and then one drop of flurbiprofen to the right eye every 5 minutes ×3. Once the patient was prepared and draped in the usual sterile ophthalmic fashion, a limited lateral peritomy was performed.

Hemostasis was achieved with bipolar cautery and then a keratome was used to enter the eye. Healon GV was placed in the eye to maintain anterior chamber formation.

A super-sharp blade was used to make a paracentesis at 6 o'clock. Then a cystotome was used to make a rent in the anterior capsule. A continuous curvilinear capsulorrhexis was attempted with a capsulorrhexis forcep. However, the cataract was such that it was anterior polar in nature and it was off center. It wasn't directly on the pupillary axis. That anterior polar protrusion made it so that continuing the continuous curvilinear capsulorrhexis was impossible so a vitrector was placed in the eye. The lens was removed, including the cataract. Then Healon GV was used to inflate the eye again. A rent was made in the posterior capsule and a limited anterior vitrectomy was performed through that rent. The incision was widened with a 3.2 short cut blade and then a 27.5 diopter SA60AT single piece intraocular lens was injected into the eye, serial number 829167.075, and the lens was rotated to be in place. It was found to be in good position.

The Healon was removed with aspiration of the vitrector. The incision was closed with a double armed 8-0 Vicryl suture, mattress fashion suturing of the incision. It was found to be water tight. Then the conjunctiva was closed with one interrupted 7-0 chromic gut suture. 2.5 cc of dexamethasone was injected over the incision and then 0.4 cc of Kefzol was injected in the inferonasal quadrant.

The patient tolerated the procedure well. He received a drop of Pred Forte in his eye, followed by Betadine, followed by TobraDex. A pressure patch, followed by a shield, was then placed on his eye and held in place with Tegaderm. The patient tolerated the procedure well. He was extubated in the operating room and taken to the recovery room in satisfactory condition.

Answer Sheet

Directions: Be sure to enter all medical record codes in the manner provided in the sample below, paying special attention to the decimal placement for each code. The codes must be typed on the answer sheet in the boxes provided on the computer screen using the keyboard. A decimal point (.) has been provided as a guide for entering each ICD-9-CM code. **You will lose credit if the digits of the codes are correct, but the decimal point has been incorrectly placed.**

CASE 12 DIAGNOSES   **ICD-9-CM**

DX1				.		
DX2				.		
DX3				.		
DX4				.		

CASE 12 PROCEDURES   **CPT/HCPCS**

PR1					
PR2					
PR3					
PR4					
PR5					
PR6					

CASE STUDY 13

Please code for the services of the physician.

Practice Exam 1   CASE 13

DATE OF PROCEDURE: 11/21/20XX

PROCEDURE: 24-hour pH probe

INDICATIONS: The patient is a complicated teenager with type 1 diabetes who has had issues with delayed gastric emptying. She is a known diabetic and she does have GI reflux. She is here for full evaluation of that symptom complex and is accompanied by her mother, who has signed an informed consent.

The double-bore pH probe was placed nasally when the patient was under anesthesia. The overall Boix-Ochoa score was 24.5, with normal being less than 16.6. There was no reflux during the night when she was asleep with the exception of one very prolonged episode that lasted 26.3 minutes. The overall reflux score was 6.8% with normal being less than 5.1%.

It would be advisable for her to stay on the medication profile that she is already taking but I do not think she is a candidate for surgery.

Answer Sheet

Directions: Be sure to enter all medical record codes in the manner provided in the sample below, paying special attention to the decimal placement for each code. The codes must be typed on the answer sheet in the boxes provided on the computer screen using the keyboard. A decimal point (.) has been provided as a guide for entering each ICD-9-CM code. **You will lose credit if the digits of the codes are correct, but the decimal point has been incorrectly placed.**

CASE 13 DIAGNOSES   **ICD-9-CM**

DX1				.		
DX2				.		
DX3				.		
DX4				.		

CASE 13 PROCEDURES   **CPT/HCPCS**

PR1					
PR2					
PR3					
PR4					
PR5					
PR6					

CASE STUDY 14

Please code for the services of the physician and the office.

Practice Exam 1   CASE 14

DATE OF PROCEDURE: 03/07/20XX

HISTORY: This is a 59-year-old man with metastatic lung cancer who presented for EEG in the office with a diagnosis of status epilepticus on March 3, 20XX.

CONDITIONS: This is an 18-channel EEG done using the 10–20 system electrode placement. During the study, the patient was not able to follow commands and at times he groaned and yawned throughout this examination.

FINDINGS: The EEG begins with the patient's eyes closed and there is a posterior dominant rhythm of 7 on the left and 7 on the right. Photic stimulation and hyperventilation were not done. Sleep was not obtained. There was some left temporal slowing shown in leads T5-01 and FP1-F3. There was no epileptiform activity seen.

IMPRESSION: This is an abnormal EEG due to the slowing seen on the left temporofrontal area.

Answer Sheet

Directions: Be sure to enter all medical record codes in the manner provided in the sample below, paying special attention to the decimal placement for each code. The codes must be typed on the answer sheet in the boxes provided on the computer screen using the keyboard. A decimal point (.) has been provided as a guide for entering each ICD-9-CM code. **You will lose credit if the digits of the codes are correct, but the decimal point has been incorrectly placed.**

CASE 14 DIAGNOSES   **ICD-9-CM**

					.		
DX1					.		
DX2					.		
DX3					.		
DX4					.		

CASE 14 PROCEDURES   **CPT/HCPCS**

PR1					
PR2					
PR3					
PR4					
PR5					
PR6					

CASE STUDY 15

Please code for the services of the physician.

Practice Exam 1 ## CASE 15

The patient, age 2 years, was seen today in the office for a brainstem auditory evoked response (BAER) evaluation and an evoked otoacoustic emissions (EOAE) evaluation. The following history was obtained upon review of the hospital medical record, and her parents' report: She has a diagnosis of Klippel-Feil anomaly, Sprengel deformity, and ventricular septal defect. She is currently receiving speech therapy services at the Little Red School House. Reportedly, she passed her newborn hearing screening. She was seen for behavioral testing on 9/15/20XX, although could not be conditioned to behavioral testing techniques. She is being seen today to establish her current hearing status and to rule out hearing difficulties as contributing to her developmental speech delay.

OTOLOGIC EVALUATION: Prior to today's hearing evaluation, her ears were examined and both of her ears were clear of any middle ear involvement.

BAER EVALUATION: Today's evaluation was completed in the PACU under general anesthesia. The patient was monitored throughout by an anesthesiologist. A four-electrode array was utilized in conjunction with both one- and two-channel recordings. Please note that the BAER evaluation does not assess how an individual will use his or her hearing, but rather it is a measure of neural synchrony along the auditory pathway.

CLICK-EVOKED BAER: Stimulus parameters included monaural presentation of alternating polarity click stimuli presented at a rate of 39.1/s via insert earphones with 1,000+ clicks average per run. It is important to note that the click-evoked BAER typically does not assess hearing acuity below 2,000 Hz.

A Wave V was recorded at 40 and 25 dBnHL for the right ear and at 40 and 20 dBnHL for the left ear. No replicable neural response was observed at 20 dBnHL for the right ear. Absolute Wave V latencies were within normal limits when compared with age-appropriate norms at each stimulus level for both ears. Waveform morphology was good. These results suggest borderline normal peripheral hearing sensitivity for the right ear and normal peripheral hearing sensitivity for the left ear, typically somewhere within the 2,000 to 4,000 Hz frequency range.

TONE-PIP EVOKED BAER: Stimulus parameters included monaural presentation of 500, 1,000, 2,000, and 4,000 Hz rarefaction polarity tone pip stimuli at a rate of 39.1/s via insert earphones with 1,000+ tone pips averaged per run.

Visual detection thresholds for both ears were established at 20 dBnHL at 500, 1,000, 2,000, and 4,000 Hz. These results are consistent with normal periphery hearing sensitivity across a broad frequency range for both ears.

EOAE EVALUATION: She was also evaluated for evoked otoacoustic emissions using the ILO 88 hardware and software. EOAEs are acoustic signals generated by the cochlea in response to external auditory stimulation.

They are a physiologically vulnerable indicator of cochlear status, specifically, outer hair cells. In response to click stimuli, EOAEs provide information over a broad frequency range (about 505,000 Hz). EOAE generation is independent of neural activity, and thus, measures cochlear status independent of CNS status. In response to click stimuli at approximately 80 to 86 dBpeSPL, emissions were present from about 1,875 to 5,429 Hz for the right ear and from about 1,406 to 4,804 Hz for the left ear. Notably, the evoked otoacoustic emissions recordings were rather noisy due to acoustic noise levels of the test environment. These results are suggestive of at least near-normal hearing sensitivity for the aforementioned frequency ranges in both ears.

SUMMARY AND RECOMMENDATIONS: Today's test results were discussed with the patient's parents in the context of the Audiogram of Familiar Sounds. The patient has normal peripheral hearing sensitivity across a broad frequency range for both ears. We have ruled out hearing loss as contributing to her speech and language development. However, given her diagnosis of Klippel-Feil anomaly and its association with hearing loss, it is recommended that we retest her hearing using behavioral test methods in approximately 1 year or sooner if concerns arise.

Answer Sheet

Directions: Be sure to enter all medical record codes in the manner provided in the sample below, paying special attention to the decimal placement for each code. The codes must be typed on the answer sheet in the boxes provided on the computer screen using the keyboard. A decimal point (.) has been provided as a guide for entering each ICD-9-CM code. **You will lose credit if the digits of the codes are correct, but the decimal point has been incorrectly placed.**

CASE 15 DIAGNOSES   **ICD-9-CM**

DX1				.		
DX2				.		
DX3				.		
DX4				.		

CASE 15 PROCEDURES   **CPT/HCPCS**

PR1					
PR2					
PR3					
PR4					
PR5					
PR6					

CASE STUDY 16

*Please code for the services
of the physician (professional)
and the technical component (total service).*

Practice Exam 1   CASE 16

REASON FOR EXAMINATION: Fourth nerve palsy

RESULTS:

CLINICAL HISTORY: Left fourth nerve palsy

EXAMINATION: MRI brain with and without contrast 1/18/20XX

COMPARISON: None

TECHNIQUE: Thin section axial T1, axial T2, T2, FLAIR, diffusion, ADC, and coronal T2, T1. Postcontrast T1 axial, Thin section T1, sagittal, and coronal. 3 cc of gadolinium was used.

Sedation was provided by anesthesia.

FINDINGS: No midline shift. No mass in the brain or brainstem. No abnormal signal in the brainstem. No abnormal signal or enhancement in the expected course of the fourth cranial nerves. Mild prominence of the supratentorial subarachnoid spaces. Third ventricle is mildly prominent. Lateral and fourth ventricles are normal. No mass or obstructing lesion in the aqueduct or tectum.

There are two ovoid, cystic foci in the periventricular white matter measuring 10 mm × 3 mm adjacent to the atria of the left lateral ventricle, likely prominent perivascular spaces.

No evidence of acute infarct on diffusion-weighted sequences.

No Chiari malformation. Normal corpus callosum. Normal myelination for age.

The paranasal sinuses and orbits are normal. There is diffuse high T2 signal in the mastoid air cells.

IMPRESSION:

1. Fourth cranial nerve palsy. No mass or abnormal signal in the brainstem. No abnormal signal or enhancement in the expected course of the fourth cranial nerves.

2. Mild prominence of the supratentorial subarachnoid spaces with mildly enlarged third ventricle and normal lateral and fourth ventricles. No obstructing mass identified, although communicating hydrocephalus could have this appearance.

Answer Sheet

Directions: Be sure to enter all medical record codes in the manner provided in the sample below, paying special attention to the decimal placement for each code. The codes must be typed on the answer sheet in the boxes provided on the computer screen using the keyboard. A decimal point (.) has been provided as a guide for entering each ICD-9-CM code. **You will lose credit if the digits of the codes are correct, but the decimal point has been incorrectly placed.**

CASE 16 DIAGNOSES   **ICD-9-CM**

DX1				.		
DX2				.		
DX3				.		
DX4				.		

CASE 16 PROCEDURES   **CPT/HCPCS**

PR1						
PR2						
PR3						
PR4						
PR5						
PR6						

Practice Exam 2
Multiple Choice Questions

Domain 1: Health Information Documentation

1. The coder notes that the physician has prescribed Retrovir for the patient. The coder might find which of the following on the patient's discharge summary?

    a. Otitis media

    b. AIDS

    c. Toxic shock syndrome

    d. Bacteremia

2. What diagnosis would the coder expect to see when a patient with pneumonia has inhaled food, liquid, or oil?

    a. Lobar pneumonia

    b. *Pneumocystis carinii* pneumonia

    c. Interstitial pneumonia

    d. Aspiration pneumonia

3. Where would a coder who needed to locate the histology of a documented breast cancer most likely find this information?

    a. Pathology report

    b. Progress notes

    c. Nurse's notes

    d. Operative report

4. A physician sees a patient for congestive heart failure. The patient is known to have a hiatal hernia and arthritis. The congestive heart failure is evaluated, blood pressure recorded, and medications adjusted for the congestive heart failure and the hypertension. What conditions are reportable?

    a. Congestive heart failure

    b. Congestive heart failure; hypertension

    c. Congestive heart failure; hypertension; arthritis

    d. Congestive heart failure; hypertension; arthritis; hiatal hernia

5. A patient is evaluated by his family practitioner for acute chest pain. The physician documents as the final diagnosis chest pain due to probable gastric ulcer and a history of cholecystectomy. What should the coder report?

   a. Chest pain; gastric ulcer

   b. Gastric ulcer

   c. Chest pain

   d. Chest pain; history of cholecystectomy

6. The coder notes that on the patient's laboratory results, the hemoglobin is 7.3 g/dL. The physician orders iron supplements. What should the coder report?

   a. Abnormal laboratory findings

   b. Iron-deficiency anemia

   c. Hemorrhaging

   d. The coder should query the physician to ask him to add an appropriate diagnosis

7. Where would information on treatment given on a particular encounter be found in the health record?

   a. Problem list

   b. Physician's orders

   c. Progress notes

   d. Physical examination

8. The patient's vital signs are part of which type of data in the health record?

   a. Medical history

   b. Physical examination

   c. Demographic data

   d. Physician's orders

Domain 2: ICD-9-CM Diagnosis Coding

9. In ICD-9-CM, this symbol is used to enclose synonyms, alternative wordings, abbreviations, and explanatory phrases:

   a. Square brackets

   b. Parentheses

   c. Slanted brackets

   d. Brace

10. The use of this symbol simplifies ICD-9-CM tabular entries and saves printing space by reducing repetitive wording and connects a series of terms on the left or right with a statement on the opposite side. This symbol is a:

    a. Section mark

    b. Lozenge

    c. Colon

    d. Brace

11. In ICD-9-CM, the fifth digit subclassification used with categories V30–V39 indicates whether a baby was:

    a. Born outside the hospital and not hospitalized

    b. Born in hospital and whether or not it was a Cesarean delivery

    c. Born at home

    d. Born before admission to hospital

12. Which of the following would be classified to an ICD-9-CM category for viral diseases?

    a. Chlamydia

    b. Streptococcus

    c. Epstein-Barr

    d. *Candida albicans*

13. Symptomatic HIV infection should be coded to which of the following codes:

    a. 795.71: Nonspecific serologic evidence of human immunodeficiency virus (HIV)

    b. 042: Human immunodeficiency virus (HIV) disease

    c. V69.8: Other problems related to lifestyle

    d. V08: Asymptomatic HIV infection

14. Which of the following conditions would be considered a late effect?

    a. Scarring following a third-degree burn

    b. Polycystic kidney disease

    c. Medication taken by the wrong person

    d. Pathologic fracture of the vertebra due to osteoporosis

15. A patient is admitted with first-, second-, and third-degree burns of the back. How would this be coded?

    a. Code second-degree burn only

    b. Code all the first-, second-, and third-degree burns

    c. Code first-degree burn only

    d. Code third-degree burn only

16. In ICD-9-CM, burns are classified in Category 948 according to the extent of body surface involved. What principle/rule is involved in estimating this body surface?

   a. Code only any third-degree burns

   b. Code burns as a late effect

   c. Code according to the rule of nines

   d. Code burns as multiple burns

17. According to ICD-9-CM, an adverse effect of a medication taken in conjunction with an alcoholic beverage is to be coded as a(n):

   a. Late effect

   b. Poisoning

   c. Complication

   d. Adverse reaction

18. In ICD-9-CM, which one of the following conditions is a mechanical complication of an internal implant, device, or graft?

   a. Scarring due to presence of breast implants

   b. Inflammation due to indwelling catheter

   c. Pain due to renal dialysis device

   d. Obstruction of heart valve prostheses

19. The diagnosis of "allergic reaction to unknown drug" would be considered to be a(n):

   a. Adverse effect

   b. Late effect

   c. Poisoning

   d. Misadventure

20. A patient presents to the physician's office after a fall from a chair. The patient is complaining of pain in the right leg so the physician orders an x-ray. The final impression was: Simple greenstick fracture, shafts of tibia and fibula. How would this be coded?

   a. 823.02: Fracture of tibia and fibula, upper end, closed

   b. 823.32: Fracture of tibia and fibula, shaft, open

   c. 823.90: Fracture of tibia, unspecified part, open

   d. 823.22: Fracture of tibia and fibula, shaft, closed

21. The patient is a 5-year-old girl whose clothes caught fire while she was helping her mother bake cookies at home. She suffered first- and second-degree burns of her abdomen and right arm. The physician dressed the burns and prescribed antibiotics. Impression: Burns of her abdomen and right arm. How would this be coded?

942.1 Burn of trunk, erythema
942.2 Burn of trunk, blisters, epidermal loss
942.3 Burn of trunk, full-thickness skin loss, NOS

    Fifth Digit Subclassification for use with Category 942:
        0—trunk, unspecified site
        1—breast
        2—chest wall, excluding breast and nipple
        3—abdominal wall
        4—back (any part)
        5—genitalia
        9—other and multiple sites of trunk

943.1 Burn of upper limb, except wrist and hand, erythema
943.2 Burn of upper limb, except wrist and hand, blisters, epidermal loss
943.3 Burn of upper limb, except wrist and hand, full-thickness skin loss, NOS

    Fifth Digit Subclassification for use with Category 943:
        0—upper limb, unspecified site
        1—forearm
        2—elbow
        3—upper arm
        4—axilla
        5—shoulder
        6—scapular region
        9—multiple sites of upper limb, except wrist and hand

---

a. 942.33; 943.31

b. 943.20; 942.23

c. 943.13; 942.10

d. 942.33; 943.20

22. A female patient is seen in the physician's office because of pain in her right lower leg. The leg was also red and swollen. The physician was concerned because the patient was postoperative and after a careful examination, rendered the final impression of: Post-operative cellulitis of right lower leg.

682.6	Other cellulitis and abscess, leg, except foot
682.7	Other cellulitis and abscess, foot, except toes
682.8	Other cellulitis and abscess, other specified sites
998.31	Disruption of internal operation (surgical) wound
998.32	Disruption of external operation (surgical) wound
998.51	Postoperative infection, infected postoperative seroma
998.59	Postoperative infection, other postoperative infection

   a. 998.59; 682.8

   b. 998.59; 682.6

   c. 682.6; 998.31

   d. 682.7; 998.51

Domain 3: CPT and HCPCS II Coding

23. A Medicare patient with a family history of colon cancer and a personal history of colon polyps undergoes an examination of the entire colon and the terminal ileum. What is the correct coding assignment for this procedure?

   a. G0104: Colorectal cancer screening, flexible sigmoidoscopy

   b. G0105: Colorectal cancer screening, colonoscopy on individual at high risk

   c. 45300: Sigmoidoscopy, flexible; diagnostic, with or without collection of specimen(s) by brushing or washing

   d. 45378: Colonoscopy, flexible, proximal to splenic flexure; diagnostic, with or without collection of specimen(s) by brushing or washing, with or without colon decompression

24. The following coding was reviewed by the coding manager before the claims were submitted. What change would the coding manager request to help ensure payment?

Case	CPT Code(s)	Description	Diagnosis	Description
1	90713	Polio vaccine	V04.81	Influenza vaccine
2	82465 73030	Cholesterol Shoulder x-ray	719.41 272.0	Shoulder pain Hypercholesterolemia

   a. Modifiers should be placed on the CPT codes

   b. Code the diagnoses codes to a greater level of specificity

   c. Additional CPT codes are required to describe the service

   d. Link the diagnoses codes correctly to the procedures

25. What is the proper code assignment when the documentation states simple wound repair of three arm lacerations at 1.5 cm, 3.0 cm, and 4.0 cm and intermediate wound repair of two hand lacerations at 1.5 cm and 2.0 cm?

12001	Simple repair of superficial wounds of scalp, neck, axillae, external genitalia, trunk and/or extremities (including hands and feet); 2.5 cm or less	
12002	2.6 cm to 7.5 cm	
12004	7.6 cm to 12.5 cm	
12005	12.6 cm to 20.0 cm	
12041	Repair, intermediate, wounds of neck, hands, feet and/or external genitalia; 2.5 cm or less	
12042	2.6 cm to 7.5 cm	
12044	7.6 cm to 12.5 cm	

a. 12004, 12042

b. 12044

c. 12005

d. 12001, 12002, 12002, 12041, 12041

26. When the physician's office performs a bilateral hand x-ray and the physician interprets the x-ray, what modifier(s) are required on the claim?

–26	Professional component
–50	Bilateral
–51	Multiple procedure
–LT	Left side
–RT	Right side
–TC	Technical component

a. –50

b. –TC, –51

c. –LT, –RT

d. –26, –LT, –RT

27. The physician excises two benign lesions measuring 0.5 cm and 2.0 cm from the patient's shoulder. Each excision site was closed with a simple repair. How should the coder code this service?

a. Code the excision of a 2.5 cm lesion

b. Code the excision of a 2.5 cm lesion and a 2.5 cm simple repair

c. Code the excision of a 0.5 cm lesion and a 2.0 cm lesion

d. Code the excision of each lesion separately and the simple repairs separately

28. Chemotherapy is provided at the physician's office for a patient with colorectal cancer. The patient receives 5-Fu over 38 minutes and oxaliplatin over 42 minutes for chemotherapy and a nonchemotherapy drug, leucovorin, for 5 minutes. How is this infusion service coded?

96413	Chemotherapy administration, intravenous infusion technique; up to 1 hour, single or initial substance/drug
96415	each additional hour (List separately in addition to code for primary procedure)
96417	each additional sequential infusion (different substance/drug), up to 1 hour (List separately in addition to code for primary procedure)
96365	Intravenous infusion, for therapy, prophylaxis, or diagnosis (specify substance or drug); initial, up to 1 hour
96374	Therapeutic, prophylactic or diagnostic injection (specify substance or drug); intravenous push, single or initial substance/drug

   a. 96413, 96365

   b. 96413, 96415, 96374

   c. 96413, 96417

   d. 96413, 96417, 96374

29. The patient complains of pain, swelling, and the feeling of warmth in the ankle. The physician aspirates 12 cc of fluid from a cyst in the patient's ankle joint. How is this procedure coded?

   a. 10021: Fine needle aspiration; without imaging guidance

   b. 20605: Arthrocentesis, aspiration and/or injection; intermediate joint or bursa (for example, temporomandibular, acromioclavicular, wrist, elbow, or ankle, olecranon bursa)

   c. 20615: Aspiration and injection for treatment of bone cyst

   d. 27604: Incision and drainage, leg or ankle; infected bursa

30. The CPT book tells coders that a code description has changed from last year by preceding the code with which of the following symbols?

   a. •

   b. ▲

   c. > <

   d. +

31. The following is a summary of visits for John Smith on November 2:

> 9:30 a.m. Seen by Dr. X for asthma, requiring nebulizer treatment and medication
>
> 3:30 p.m. Seen by Dr. X again for worsening asthma, requiring another nebulizer treatment and more medication

To help ensure payment, which of the following modifiers should be reported by Dr. X for the services provided at 3:30 p.m.?

a. –51: Multiple procedures

b. –58: Staged or related procedure or service by the same physician during the postoperative period

c. –76: Repeat procedure by same physician

d. –77: Repeat procedure by another physician

32. Which of the following is excluded from the surgical global:

a. Consultation to determine the need for procedure

b. Local, regional, or topical anesthesia administered

c. The surgical procedure performed

d. Routine postoperative follow-up care

33. The pathologist does a gross and microscopic examination on three surgical specimens from a bronchoscopy procedure. Specimens submitted were biopsies of lung, bronchus, and trachea. The pathologist is not employed by the hospital. What is the correct code assignment for the services of the pathologist?

88300	Level I—Surgical pathology, gross examination only
88305	Level IV—Surgical pathology, gross and microscopic examination
–26	Professional component
–TC	Technical component

a. 88300, 88305

b. 88305–26

c. 88305–26 ×3

d. 88300–TC, 88300–TC, 88305–TC

34. The patient (not covered by Medicare) is sent to a dermatologist by her primary care physician for diagnosis of a suspicious rash. A detailed history and examination are done, a biopsy is taken, and medication is prescribed. The findings are sent back to the primary care physician. How is this E/M service coded?

    a. 99203: Office or other outpatient visit for the evaluation and management of a new patient, which requires these three key components of detailed history, detailed examination, and medical decision making of low complexity.

    b. 99214: Office or other outpatient visit for the evaluation and management of an established patient, which requires at least two of these three key components of detailed history, detailed examination, and medical decision making of moderate complexity.

    c. 99243: Office consultation for a new or established patient, which requires these three key components of detailed history, detailed examination, and medical decision making of low complexity.

    d. 99254: Inpatient consultation for a new or established patient, which requires three key components of comprehensive history, comprehensive examination, and medical decision making of moderate complexity.

35. A portion of a patient's kidney is removed using an incisional technique. How is this service coded?

    a. 50045: Nephrotomy, with exploration

    b. 50240: Nephrectomy, partial

    c. 50340: Recipient nephrectomy (separate procedure)

    d. 50543: Laparoscopy, surgical; partial nephrectomy

36. The patient has a misaligned phalangeal shaft fracture demonstrated on a two-view x-ray, performed and read by the physician in the office. The physician manipulates the finger into alignment and places a rigid finger splint. How are these services coded?

26720	Closed treatment of phalangeal shaft fracture, proximal or middle phalanx, finger or thumb; without manipulation, each
26725	with manipulation, with or without skin or skeletal traction, each
26727	Percutaneous skeletal fixation of unstable phalangeal shaft fracture, proximal or middle phalanx, finger or thumb, with manipulation, each
73120	Radiologic examination, hand; 2 views
73140	Radiologic examination, finger(s), minimum of 2 views

    a. 26720, 73120

    b. 26725, 73120

    c. 26725, 73140

    d. 26727, 73140

Domain 4: Reimbursement

37. Which term describes the linking of every procedure or service provided to a patient to a diagnosis that justifies the need for performing the service?

    a. Medical necessity

    b. Managed care

    c. Medical decision-making

    d. Level of services

38. Which payment system was introduced in 1992 and replaced Medicare's customary, prevailing, and reasonable (CPR) payment system?

    a. Diagnosis-related groups

    b. Resource-based relative value scale system

    c. Long-term care drugs

    d. Resource utilization groups

39. Which report should be consulted to determine the most frequently used CPT codes to be placed on the physician's charge ticket?

    a. Revenue production

    b. Service mix

    c. Service distribution

    d. Case mix

40. What tool could be used to evaluate utilization patterns for Evaluation and Management (E/M) codes as illustrated here?

Month	CPT Code	Description	Qty	Charge	Reimbursement	Projected Revenue
June	99215	Estab Pt. Comp	79	$125.00	$100.00	$7,900.00
June	99211	Nurse only	334	$35.00	$24.50	$8,183.00
June	99212	Estab Pt. Problem	412	$40.00	$32.00	$13,184.00
June	99214	Estab Pt. Detailed	234	$80.00	$64.00	$14,976.00
June	99213	Estab Pt. Expanded	759	$50.00	$40.00	$30,360.00

    a. Missed charges report

    b. Service distribution report

    c. Service mix report

    d. Diagnosis distribution report

41. Which of the following is the practice of coding/charging one or two middle levels of service exclusively for all patient encounters?

   a. Clustering

   b. Unbundling

   c. Optimizing

   d. Inappropriate linking of codes

42. What is a claim called that contains all required data elements needed to process and pay the claim quickly?

   a. Open

   b. Clean

   c. Closed

   d. Final

43. The amount that a nonparticipating (non-PAR) physician who does not accept assignment can bill a Medicare beneficiary is called the:

   a. Non-PAR value

   b. Contractual limit

   c. Limiting charge

   d. Nonassigned charge

44. A coder uses local coverage determinations (LCDs) from Medicare to identify:

   a. What procedures require prior approval before payment is made by the third party

   b. What CPT codes justify the necessity of a test or service

   c. What is the reimbursement for a specific procedure

   d. What ICD-9-CM codes justify the medical necessity of a test or service

Domain 5: Data Quality and Analysis

45. After reviewing the following hospital charges for Dr. Peters for patient #213429, the coder should:

Patient #213429

Date of Admission: 8/12/20XX

Date of Discharge: 8/15/20XX

Date of Service	CPT Code	Description	Diagnosis	Charge
8/12/20XX	99255	Consultation	345.10	$247.00
8/13/20XX	99221	Initial hospital	401.9	$167.00
8/14/20XX	99221	Initial hospital	345.10	$167.00
8/15/20XX	99238	Hospital discharge	401.9	$105.00

   a. Question that a different diagnosis was used on some days

   b. Bill the codes exactly as the physician submitted them

   c. Notice that the two daily visits are coded incorrectly

   d. Request the records from the hospital to verify the services

46. Once an audit has been completed, what should the coding manager do?

   a. Perform another audit in six months before doing any education

   b. Provide education about the results and then perform a follow-up audit

   c. Make sure that no one finds out the results of the audit to maintain privacy and security

   d. Report the audit findings to the Office of the Inspector General as required by the Compliance Plan

47. What is the best tool to use when completing a yearly update of office encounter forms?

   a. Appendix A of the CPT book

   b. Appendix B of the CPT book

   c. The CMS Web site (cms.hhs.gov)

   d. An educational text about CPT

48. The coding manager completes an audit of patients who were listed on the surgery schedule for cervical two-level discectomies. After reviewing this coded data, what education did the manager determine would be beneficial for the coding staff?

| 63030 | Laminotomy (hemilaminectomy), with decompression of nerve root(s), including partial facetectomy, foraminotomy and/or excision of herniated intervertebral disc, including open or endoscopically-assisted approaches; 1 interspace, lumbar |
| 63035 | each additional interspace, cervical or lumbar (List separately in addition to code for primary procedure.) |

Case	CPT Code	Diagnosis	Description
1	63030	722.0	Displacement of cervical intervertebral disc
	63035	722.0	Displacement of cervical intervertebral disc
2	63030	722.71	Intervertebral disc disorder with myelopathy
	63035	722.71	Intervertebral disc disorder with myelopathy
3	63030	839.04	Dislocation, fourth cervical vertebra (traumatic)
	63035	839.04	Dislocation, fourth cervical vertebra (traumatic)

a. Linking of diagnoses to procedures

b. ICD-9-CM coding for specificity

c. The use of add-on codes

d. Anatomy of the spinal column

49. If the physician documents "Counseling, 20 minutes on attention deficit disorder" and wants to assign code 99213, what additional documentation must be made to allow this code assignment?

a. The nature of the presenting problem

b. The history component of the documentation

c. The examination component of the documentation

d. The length of the entire visit

50. A 60-year-old woman calls the office saying that she was billed for a contraceptive shot, which "could not be right." The claim for that date shows 1 unit of J1055 was billed, with diagnoses of V07.4 and 627.3. The encounter form for the visit states "Estrogen therapy" but the documentation does not show that an injection was given. What error does the coding manager suspect?

> J1051 Injection, medroxyprogesterone acetate (conjugated estrogen), 50 mg
>
> J1055 Injection, medroxyprogesterone acetate (conjugated estrogen) for contraceptive use, 150 mg
>
> V07.4 Postmenopausal hormone replacement therapy
>
> 627.3 Postmenopausal atrophic vaginitis

   a. The coder chose a code for the wrong medication

   b. The coder chose a code for the wrong dosage of medication

   c. The coder assumed that estrogen was administered at that visit

   d. The coder reported an incorrect diagnosis code for the service

Domain 6: Information and Communication Technologies

51. Which of the following would be considered an advantage of using e-mail for transmission of data?

   a. Employers and online services retain the right to archive messages transmitted through their systems.

   b. E-mail may be discoverable for legal purposes.

   c. E-mail can be used to clarify treatment instructions or medication administration.

   d. E-mail can be printed, circulated, forwarded, and stored in numerous paper and electronic files.

52. The physician asks that a computerized record be kept of all his patients with basic demographic and encounter data compiled. What software application would be used?

   a. Word processing

   b. Database

   c. Spreadsheet

   d. Process tracking

53. Which of the following software applications would be used to aid in the coding function in a physician's office?

   a. Grouper

   b. Encoder

   c. Pricer

   d. Diagnosis calculator

54. A physician asks that his total patient encounters be calculated by month, by quarter, and by year. The physician would also like a monthly average. What software application should be used?

   a. Word processing

   b. Database

   c. Spreadsheet

   d. Process tracking

Domain 7: Compliance and Regulatory Issues

55. The term that refers to the degree to which the same results are achieved each time a record is coded during a coding audit is:

   a. Validity

   b. Completeness

   c. Reliability

   d. Timeliness

56. The term used to describe private citizens who may bring suit on behalf of themselves and the government against fraudulent healthcare providers is:

   a. Defendants

   b. Qui tam plaintiffs

   c. Res ipsa loquitor

   d. Res gestae

57. The head of the surgery department asks to see a patient's medical record. This physician is not listed as her surgeon in the record. What do you do?

   a. Give the physician the medical record as he requested

   b. Inform the physician that because he is not listed as the patient's surgeon he must obtain the appropriate authorization signed by the patient in order to review the record

   c. Inform the physician that you are unable to provide the chart because he is not listed as the patient's attending physician

   d. Inform the physician that you are too busy to retrieve the patient's chart

58. A child was examined and treated for child abuse in the Emergency Department at the hospital. As a result, the child has been taken into protective custody by the Office of Child Protection because of suspected child abuse by the parents. The father requests copies of the designated record set for the visit. He has a copy of the child's birth certificate listing him as the father and he possesses a picture ID. Do you release a copy of the Emergency Department record?

   a. Yes, after he has completed a legitimate release of information authorization.

   b. Decline to release the information and contact the hospital's attorney.

   c. Contact the Office of Child Protection for permission to release the record.

   d. Refer the matter to the hospital administrator and follow the administration's instructions after he meets with the father.

59. The "minimum necessary rule" refers to which of the following:

    a. Copying all billing and medical records as requested by the patient

    b. Releasing copies of the entire medical record for all disclosure requests

    c. Disclosing personal health information is held to the smallest amount of information necessary to accomplish the intended purpose of the use or disclosure

    d. Requesting personal health information by public officials who have a right to the information as dictated by state law

60. Although the HIPAA Privacy Rule allows patients access to personal health information about themselves, which of the following cannot be disclosed to patients?

    a. Interpretation of x-rays by the radiologist

    b. Billing records

    c. Progress notes written by the attending physician

    d. Psychotherapy notes

Practice Exam 2 Medical Cases

CASE STUDY 1

Please code for the services of the physician.

Practice Exam 2   CASE 1

ESTABLISHED PATIENT

HISTORY OF PRESENT ILLNESS: The patient is a 7-year-old boy who presents today with his mother due to jamming his finger in the door this morning. He caught his right middle finger in the door leading to his garage. It occurred about 40 minutes prior to his arrival at the clinic.

PHYSICAL EXAMINATION: Temperature 98.4, pulse 79, respirations 14, blood pressure 90/60. Heart has a regular rate and rhythm. Lungs are clear to auscultation. Abdomen is soft. The patient is alert and resting on his back on the examination table. Examination of the right middle finger shows some swelling and a flap of skin to the distal right middle finger that is raised. There appears to be no involvement of the nail bed itself, no subungual hematoma present. Distal extremity is neurovascularly intact.

RADIOGRAPHS: X-rays done on the right middle finger done at the imaging center do not demonstrate any fracture to the distal tip. Await official report of radiology.

PROCEDURE: The patient was taken to the procedure room. Informed consent was obtained from the patient's mother and she gave permission for laceration repair. He was placed in a supine position and a digital block was performed with 2 mL of 2% lidocaine. The area was then cleansed and irrigated with copious amounts of sterile saline. The area was then draped in a sterile fashion and three 5-0 Ethilon interrupted sutures were placed to realign the 1-cm flap. Dressing was applied and patient tolerated it well.

ASSESSMENT: Laceration of the right middle finger

PLAN:

1. Status post repair.

2. Wound care directions were given. The patient will follow up in 7 to 10 days for suture removal or sooner if any condition worsens or problems arise.

HISTORY: Problem-focused

EXAMINATION: Detailed

MEDICAL DECISION-MAKING: Low

Answer Sheet

Directions: Be sure to enter all medical record codes in the manner provided in the sample below, paying special attention to the decimal placement for each code. The codes must be typed on the answer sheet in the boxes provided on the computer screen using the keyboard. A decimal point (.) has been provided as a guide for entering each ICD-9-CM code. **You will lose credit if the digits of the codes are correct, but the decimal point has been incorrectly placed.**

CASE 1 DIAGNOSES   **ICD-9-CM**

DX1				.		
DX2				.		
DX3				.		
DX4				.		

CASE 1 PROCEDURES   **CPT/HCPCS**

PR1						
PR2						
PR3						
PR4						
PR5						
PR6						

CASE STUDY 2

Please code for the services of the physician.

Practice Exam 2   CASE 2

REQUESTING PHYSICIAN: Dr. X

CONSULTING PHYSICIAN: Dr. Y

REGARDING: Hematochezia

HISTORY OF PRESENT ILLNESS: A 77-year-old white woman transferred from XYZ Medical Center on 1/6/20XX with interstitial pneumonitis. Hospital course here has been complicated by hypoxemia, renal insufficiency, and steroid-induced diabetes mellitus. The patient reports having episodes of small volume painless hematochezia at home secondary to hemorrhoids. Last evening and this morning experienced larger volume bright red blood per rectum. She has been experiencing problems with constipation. The patient reports having colonoscopy roughly 3 years ago performed elsewhere revealing diverticulosis and her aforementioned hemorrhoids. She does state that she has had sequential colonoscopies performed in the past. However, she is unclear on the findings.

PAST MEDICAL HISTORY:

1. Rheumatoid arthritis
2. Chronic renal insufficiency
3. Hypertension
4. Dyslipidemia
5. Hypothyroidism
6. Status post hysterectomy, status post appendectomy, status post back surgery, status post bilateral total knee replacements

CURRENT MEDICATIONS:

1. Coumadin
2. Novolog
3. Insulin
4. Fosamax
5. Aspirin
6. Prednisone
7. Valtrex
8. Lasix
9. Synthroid
10. Protonix
11. Zocor
12. Doxepin
13. Norvasc
14. Calcium

ALLERGIES: No known drug allergies.

FAMILY HISTORY: Negative for significant GI disease or malignancy.

SOCIAL HISTORY: Denies alcohol or tobacco use.

REVIEW OF SYSTEMS: Negative for epistaxis, hemoptysis, hematuria, history of vaginal bleeding, liver disease. All others negative.

PHYSICAL EXAMINATION:

GENERAL: She is alert and oriented in no acute distress. Chronically ill-appearing.

VITAL SIGNS: BP is 130/70, pulse is 100

INTEGUMENT: Reveals multiple scattered ecchymosis and purpura. Positive for edema, anicteric.

HEENT: Eyes—sclerae white, conjunctivae pink, nares patent without epistaxis or discharge. Oral cavity reveals some erosions at the edges of her mouth. Buccal mucosa is without significant ulcerations. Oropharynx was clear. No obvious hemorrhage.

NECK: Supple, nontender without masses, lymphadenopathy, thyromegaly.

LUNGS: Unlabored, respiration fields are clear

CARDIAC: S1, S2, regular rate and rhythm

ABDOMEN: Positive bowel sounds, soft, nontender without masses or hepato-splenomegaly

RECTAL: Her perineum is diffusely stained with blood. She does have some obvious external hemorrhage. Digital examination was painful for the patient with blood coating on the fingertip. No obvious masses. Cannot ascertain whether or not she possibly could have a fissure.

GENITOURINARY: The introitus with some blood staining. Her laboratory studies revealed a white blood cell count of 12.6, hemoglobin 9.5, platelet count 227. BUN was 47, creatinine 1.6, PT at 28.2, INR 2.8.

IMPRESSION:

1. Hematochezia. Differential diagnoses including diverticular, proctitis, fissure, hemorrhoidsulcer, possible neoplasm. Her bleeding was exacerbated by her anticoagulation.
2. Interstitial pneumonia
3. Chronic rheumatoid arthritis
4. Chronic renal insufficiency
5. Constipation

RECOMMENDATIONS:

1. Her Coumadin currently is on hold. Colonoscopy per GI. Will follow her CBC if persistent bleeding. She may need to be reversed and consider IVC filter.

2. Continue on insulin for her steroid-induced DM.

3. Continue postoperative physical therapy for her knees.

HISTORY: Comprehensive

EXAMINATION: Comprehensive

MDM: High

Answer Sheet

Directions: Be sure to enter all medical record codes in the manner provided in the sample below, paying special attention to the decimal placement for each code. The codes must be typed on the answer sheet in the boxes provided on the computer screen using the keyboard. A decimal point (.) has been provided as a guide for entering each ICD-9-CM code. **You will lose credit if the digits of the codes are correct, but the decimal point has been incorrectly placed.**

CASE 2 DIAGNOSES   **ICD-9-CM**

DX1				.		
DX2				.		
DX3				.		
DX4				.		

CASE 2 PROCEDURES   **CPT/HCPCS**

PR1					
PR2					
PR3					
PR4					
PR5					
PR6					

CASE STUDY 3

Please code for the services of the physician.

Practice Exam 2   CASE 3

CHIEF COMPLAINT: Nosebleed

HISTORY OF PRESENT ILLNESS: The patient is a 69-year-old man who presents to the emergency department with spontaneous onset of a nosebleed at approximately midnight. The patient was awakened by a sensation in his throat that he thought was posterior nasal discharge, and subsequently discovered that in fact his nose was bleeding. He was unable to achieve hemostasis at home, and so presents to the Emergency Department. He denies prior problems with nosebleeds. He further denies any history of coagulopathy, and is not on any medications that should cause anticoagulation.

PAST MEDICAL HISTORY:

1. Hypertension
2. Depression with anxiety
3. Gastroesophageal reflux disease

PAST SURGICAL HISTORY:

1. Status post appendectomy
2. Status post perforated viscus
3. Status post laminectomy

CURRENT MEDICATIONS:

1. Rabeprazole
2. Inderal
3. Amitriptyline
4. Alprazolam

ALLERGIES:

1. OPIOID analgesics
2. TORADOL

SOCIAL HISTORY: The patient is married. Lives independently with his spouse. His primary physician is Dr. X. He does not use tobacco and denies excessive ethanol use.

FAMILY HISTORY: Negative for any coagulopathy

REVIEW OF SYSTEMS: Negative, other than those items in the HPI

PHYSICAL EXAMINATION:

VITAL SIGNS: Blood pressure 132/72, pulse 84, respiration 16, temperature is 97.8

GENERAL: The patient is awake and alert. He is nontoxic, and otherwise in no acute distress.

    HEENT: Sclerae were anicteric. The palpebral conjunctivae are pink. TMs are clear bilaterally. The oropharynx demonstrated some posterior sanguinous drainage, but otherwise was clear.

    NECK: Supple

LUNGS: Breath sounds clear and symmetric

CARDIAC: Regular S1, S2. No murmur or gallop appreciated.

ABDOMEN: Soft, nontender, without hepatosplenomegaly or mass

EXTREMITIES: No deformities, clubbing, or edema. Pulses full and symmetric throughout.

SKIN: Warm and dry. No jaundice, pallor, or cyanosis noted. No skin rashes present.

NEUROLOGIC: The patient is alert and fully oriented. Pupils equal, round, and reactive to light. The remainder of the examination is nonfocal.

EMERGENCY DEPARTMENT COURSE: A nasal clip was placed and left in place for approximately 15 minutes. Reevaluation of the patient at that time revealed moderate bleeding in the right nasal passage, but the left passage was clear. The right side was subsequently packed with cotton pledgets soaked with Parkes solution. After leaving these in place for approximately 15 minutes, the bleeding was well controlled. There was, however, a single bleeding point of an exposed vessel, which was identified. This was cauterized successfully, with good hemostasis achieved. The patient's nasal passages were subsequently swabbed with antibiotic ointment. He was observed for an additional 20 to 30 minutes, and his bleeding remained well controlled. He was subsequently discharged home in good condition.

DISCHARGE INSTRUCTIONS:

1. He was advised to avoid any aspirin, and as well, to avoid blowing his nose for 2 days.

2. He was advised to continue using Neosporin or a similar antibiotic ointment to the right nasal passage three times per day.

3. He was recommended to follow up either with an ENT physician of his choice, or Dr. X in 3 to 5 days. The patient was subsequently discharged home in good condition.

EMERGENCY DEPARTMENT DIAGNOSIS: Epistaxis

HISTORY: Comprehensive

EXAMINATION: Comprehensive

MDM: Low

Answer Sheet

Directions: Be sure to enter all medical record codes in the manner provided in the sample below, paying special attention to the decimal placement for each code. The codes must be typed on the answer sheet in the boxes provided on the computer screen using the keyboard. A decimal point (.) has been provided as a guide for entering each ICD-9-CM code. **You will lose credit if the digits of the codes are correct, but the decimal point has been incorrectly placed.**

CASE 3 DIAGNOSES   **ICD-9-CM**

					.		
DX1					.		
DX2					.		
DX3					.		
DX4					.		

CASE 3 PROCEDURES   **CPT/HCPCS**

PR1					
PR2					
PR3					
PR4					
PR5					
PR6					

CASE STUDY 4

Please code for the services of the physician.

Practice Exam 2   CASE 4

REQUESTING PHYSICIAN: Dr. Z, Primary Care

HISTORY: This is a very pleasant 63-year-old white man with multiple past medical history who is seen initially with the chief complaint of altered mental status at the nursing home. An infectious disease consult has been obtained for a possible urinary tract infection and sepsis.

SOCIAL HISTORY: The patient is a nursing home resident here.

MEDICATIONS: Avonex and Norvasc

ALLERGIES: None

REVIEW OF SYSTEMS: Pertinent for altered mental status

PHYSICAL EXAMINATION:

VITAL SIGNS: The patient is currently afebrile. Blood pressure 152/94.

GENERAL: The patient is in no distress. Alert, awake, and oriented times two.

CARDIOVASCULAR: Regular rate and rhythm. Positive S1 and S2. No murmurs.

LUNGS: Clear to auscultation. No wheezes or crackles.

ABDOMEN: Bowel sounds positive. Nontender.

EXTREMITIES: Good pulses. No edema.

LABORATORY DATA: Urinalysis positive for pyuria. Urine culture with gram-negative, anaerobic *Providencia stuartii.*

ASSESSMENT:
1. Septicemia due to *Providencia Stuartii*
2. Urinary tract infection

RECOMMENDATIONS:
1. Recommend starting the patient on Rocephin.
2. Check blood cultures times two sets.

Thank you for recommending this consultation. Please fax a copy to Dr. Z's office.

HISTORY: Detailed

EXAMINATION: Detailed

MEDICAL DECISION-MAKING: Moderate

Answer Sheet

Directions: Be sure to enter all medical record codes in the manner provided in the sample below, paying special attention to the decimal placement for each code. The codes must be typed on the answer sheet in the boxes provided on the computer screen using the keyboard. A decimal point (.) has been provided as a guide for entering each ICD-9-CM code. **You will lose credit if the digits of the codes are correct, but the decimal point has been incorrectly placed.**

CASE 4 DIAGNOSES   **ICD-9-CM**

					.		
DX1					.		
DX2					.		
DX3					.		
DX4					.		

CASE 4 PROCEDURES   **CPT/HCPCS**

PR1					
PR2					
PR3					
PR4					
PR5					
PR6					

CASE STUDY 5

Please code for the services of the physician.

Practice Exam 2 CASE 5

SERVICE: Trauma service

HPI: This patient arrived at the emergency department on 10/07/20XX at approximately 19:00. The patient is a 25-year-old Hispanic woman who is status post pedestrian versus motor vehicle collision. The patient reports a questionable loss of consciousness prior to arrival. Upon arrival the patient's prehospital blood pressure was noted to be 130/90 with prehospital heart rate of 126. The patient was in severe pain, complaining of pain mostly over the left anterior chest wall and of the left leg, and was admitted to trauma service. Upon questioning the patient denied allergies.

PAST MEDICAL HISTORY: Normal

MEDICATIONS: None

PAST SURGICAL HISTORY: Significant for removal of the gallbladder

FAMILY HISTORY: Normal

SOCIAL HISTORY: Occasional use of alcohol, approximately 2 to 3 drinks per week, but the patient denied use of tobacco or illicit drugs.

REVIEW OF SYSTEMS: No fever or fatigue; no systemic complaints. The patient's dermatologic review of systems was negative. She reports no rashes or any outstanding skin conditions. The patient's ear, nose, and throat review of systems was also unremarkable. The patient's cardiovascular, pulmonary, and gastrointestinal systems were all unremarkable with no specific complaints toward chest pain, shortness of breath, or change in bowel habits. Additionally, the patient's musculoskeletal review of systems was normal without prior history of musculoskeletal disease or weakness. The patient's genitourinary review of systems was normal with no complaints of dysuria or abnormal genitalia, or burning or itching. Psychiatric and neurologic review of systems was also unremarkable. The patient's skin was unremarkable historically but upon presentation the patient did complain of a rash and abrasion secondary to her trauma.

PRIMARY SURVEY: Clear airway that required no intervention. The patient arrived in C spine immobilization in a hard collar and backboard. The patient was found to be breathing spontaneously and unlabored.

Skin was warm, normal in color, without signs of external hemorrhage. The patient's carotid, femoral, radial, and dorsalis pedis pulses were all palpable and 2+ positive.

The patient was found to be alert, GCS approximately 14 with the only abnormality of the eyes not opening spontaneously and only to voice. Pupils were found to be reactive, 4-2, and symmetric. The patient's Glasgow coma scale upon initial evaluation in the trauma bay was that of GCS 14, the patient's total trauma score was 12. The patient had a CT scan of the head, chest, abdomen, and pelvis, as well as reconstructed views of the cervical, thoracic, and lumbar spines performed. These scans were reviewed with the doctor in the radiology department. The CT of the head was negative, with no obvious skull deformity or fracture, and no intracranial bleeding. Her chest revealed several abnormalities including a pulmonary contusion of the left upper lobe, hemopneumothorax, and depressed rib fractures at ribs 2, 3, 4, 5, and 6. The rib fractures at 4 and 5 were comminuted. Rib 6 was severely displaced and crushed inward. However, upon evaluation of the CT scan there was no evidence or indication of thoracic vascular injury. CT scan of the abdomen was unremarkable. The patient's CT scan of the pelvis revealed pubic rami fracture. The patient's cervical, thoracic, and lumbar spine images were reconstructed using the CT scan. These images revealed C spine, T spine, and L spine that were essentially without abnormality. The patient's point of care laboratory results included a hemoglobin of 14.1, sodium 143, potassium 3.6, chlorine 102, BUN 12, base excess of 2, pH 7.38, PO_2 37, PCO_2 45, lactate 1.9.

SECONDARY SURVEY: HEENT: The patient's pupils were equally round and reactive to light bilaterally, going from 4 mm to 2 mm with direct light stimulation. The patient's gaze was normal with tymphanic membranes on the right and left clear. The oropharynx was found to be clear but tender at the chin. Gag reflex was intact and inclusion was normal. Neck revealed collapsed veins with trachea midline. There was no tenderness or crepitance in the neck. The chest revealed some external bilateral upper chest abrasions. The chest wall was seen to be symmetric; however, breath sounds were found to be abnormal with decreased breath sounds, particularly in the left chest. Heart sounds were regular rate and rhythm without murmurs, rubs, or gallops. The patient was not found to have crepitance of the chest wall. However, there was severe tenderness to palpation at the left anterior chest wall. Abdomen revealed no external trauma to the abdomen, no tenderness to palpation, obese but yet normal contour to the abdomen. Abdomen was dull to percussion. Pelvis stable and nontender by examination. Genitourinary revealed no blood at the meatus and the urine pregnancy test was negative. Rectal revealed normal sphincter tone with brown stool. Spine revealed a nontender cervical, thoracic, and lumbar spine. There was no evidence of step-off deformity at any of these levels. Neuro revealed motor strength 5+/5+ in both right and left upper and lower extremities. Additionally sensory examination revealed no deficits. Vascular exam revealed 2+ radial pulses bilaterally. Additionally femoral, posterior tibial, and dorsalis pulses were all 2+ bilaterally.

ASSESSMENT: 25-year-old female involved in a pedestrian versus motor vehicle trauma. The patient suffered multiple injuries. The patient suffered rib fractures from ribs 2 to 6 on the left side. Ribs 4 and 5 on the left side were found to have the comminuted fractures with resultant hemopneumothorax and pulmonary contusion.

Rib 6 was also a severely displaced rib fracture with displacement into the thoracic cavity. Reconstructed images of the cervical, thoracic, and lumbar spines were negative. C spine showed questionable transverse fracture at level T4.

PLAN:

1. Watch respiratory status due to pulmonary insult. The patient is to receive IPPV treatments in the TICU.

3. Orthopedic consultation for the suprapubic ramus fracture.

ADDENDUM ADDED

REVISION TO ADMISSION H&P DICTATION: The patient had no evidence of fracture abnormality on her C spine on reconstructed images. Repeat, there was no abnormality on C spine, which was negative. This was cleared radiographically.

HISTORY: Comprehensive

EXAMINATION: Comprehensive

MEDICAL DECISION-MAKING: High

Answer Sheet

Directions: Be sure to enter all medical record codes in the manner provided in the sample below, paying special attention to the decimal placement for each code. The codes must be typed on the answer sheet in the boxes provided on the computer screen using the keyboard. A decimal point (.) has been provided as a guide for entering each ICD-9-CM code. **You will lose credit if the digits of the codes are correct, but the decimal point has been incorrectly placed.**

CASE 5 DIAGNOSES   **ICD-9-CM**

DX1				.		
DX2				.		
DX3				.		
DX4				.		

CASE 5 PROCEDURES   **CPT/HCPCS**

PR1					
PR2					
PR3					
PR4					
PR5					
PR6					

CASE STUDY 6

Please code for the services of the physician.

Practice Exam 2

CASE 6

CHIEF COMPLAINT: Hematuria in a new patient

HISTORY OF PRESENT ILLNESS: Patient is a 36-year-old woman who presents to my office with acute onset of hematuria within the last 6 to 8 hours. However, over the last 2 days the patient has noted urinary pressure, urinary frequency, dysuria, and chills, although she denies any true rigors. She has not had any identifiable fever. She has mild low central abdominal discomfort but has had no nausea or vomiting. She has not noted changes in her bowel habits.

PAST MEDICAL HISTORY: Notable for arthritis in her right foot. There is no history of diabetes, ischemic heart disease, or hypertension. Has a significant history of schizophrenia.

SURGICAL HISTORY: She is status post corrective surgery on her right foot, status post an operative procedure on her cervix, and status post cyst removal at her right ankle.

CURRENT MEDICATIONS: Ibuprofen p.r.n.

ALLERGIES: Noted to PENICILLIN and SULFA

SOCIAL HISTORY: The patient lives independently. She smokes approximately 1/2 pack of cigarettes per day and denies excessive ethanol use.

REVIEW OF SYSTEMS:

GENERAL: Negative for any documented fevers, but the patient does report some chills. Her p.o. intake has been normal, and no weight loss described.

GI: See HPI

GU: See HPI

GYN: No unusual vaginal discharge or bleeding. The patient is sexually active. Does not believe she is pregnant.

PHYSICAL EXAMINATION:

VITAL SIGNS: Blood pressure 111/68. Pulse is 86, Respiration is 20, Temperature is 97.8

GENERAL: The patient is awake, alert, nontoxic, in no acute distress.

HEENT: Was unremarkable

NECK: Supple

LUNGS: Breath sounds clear and symmetric.

CARDIAC: Regular S2, S2. No murmur or gallop appreciated.

ABDOMEN: Soft, nontender in the upper regions with some minimal suprapubic tenderness. There are no masses, organomegaly, or peritoneal signs present, and no tenderness present.

EXTREMITIES: No deformities, clubbing, or edema. Pulses full and symmetric throughout.

SKIN: Warm and dry. No jaundice, pallor, or cyanosis noted. No skin rash is present.

NEUROLOGIC: The patient is alert, fully oriented. Pupils equal, round, and reactive to light. The remainder of her examination is nonfocal.

A voided urine specimen was obtained for pregnancy testing and an automated urinalysis. Pregnancy test was negative, and the urinalysis demonstrated specific gravity of less than 1.005 with large occult blood and a large leukocyte esterase. Microscopy revealed 3 to 5 red blood cells were seen with greater than 100 red blood cells, and only an occasional squamous cell noted.

The results of her urinalysis and my findings and recommendations were discussed with the patient in detail. She was given Levaquin 500 mg orally in the office and a prescription for 5 additional days worth. I recommended she drink plenty of fluids. Pyridium 100 mg, 1 to 2 q. 8 hours p.r.n. was prescribed for discomfort, and two tablets of Pyridium given to the patient for her use overnight. Patient was significantly agitated due to her ongoing schizophrenia. Patient was recommended to follow up with me in 3 to 5 days if not significantly improved.

DIAGNOSES: Acute urinary tract infection. Schizophrenia.

HISTORY: Extended problem-focused

EXAMINATION: Comprehensive

MEDICAL DECISION-MAKING: Moderate

Answer Sheet

Directions: Be sure to enter all medical record codes in the manner provided in the sample below, paying special attention to the decimal placement for each code. The codes must be typed on the answer sheet in the boxes provided on the computer screen using the keyboard. A decimal point (.) has been provided as a guide for entering each ICD-9-CM code. **You will lose credit if the digits of the codes are correct, but the decimal point has been incorrectly placed.**

CASE 6 DIAGNOSES   **ICD-9-CM**

					.		
DX1					.		
DX2					.		
DX3					.		
DX4					.		

CASE 6 PROCEDURES   **CPT/HCPCS**

PR1					
PR2					
PR3					
PR4					
PR5					
PR6					

CASE STUDY 7

Please code for the services of the surgeon.

Practice Exam 2 CASE 7

PREOPERATIVE DIAGNOSIS: Degenerative osteoarthritis of the right knee with resulting genu varum deformity

POSTOPERATIVE DIAGNOSIS: Degenerative osteoarthritis of the right knee with resulting genu varum deformity

OPERATION PERFORMED: Computer-assisted navigation right total knee arthroplasty

COMPONENTS USED: Biomet Vanguard femur 67.5 mm PS, tibial tray 83 mm, 10 mm PS insert, 38 mm single peg inset patella

SURGEON:

ASSISTANT:

ANESTHESIA: Continuous spinal epidural

DRAINS: One medium OrthoPAT

COMPLICATIONS: None

DESCRIPTION OF PROCEDURE: The patient was brought to the operating room. After instillation of satisfactory CSE anesthesia and placement of Foley catheter, the right lower extremity was appropriately prepared and draped in the usual sterile fashion. The two tibial trackers were placed into the proximal tibia. Tourniquet was inflated to 300 mm Hg.

A midline incision was made centered over the patella and carried down to the quadriceps mechanism. Median parapatellar incision was fashioned. Subperiosteal dissection of proximal medial plateau of the posteromedial corner was accomplished. Distal femoral trackers were placed.

At this point, the registration process was begun. Following the surgical registration with kinematic analysis, the procedure was begun.

The distal femoral tracker was navigated into position and pinned in place and confirmed. Distal femoral cut was made and verified. The 2 sizing jig was positioned in the hybrid technique for rotation and was computer navigated. The 67.5 was selected and the anterior, posterior, condylar, and chamfer cuts were made. Following this, the remnants of the anterior cruciate ligament and medial and lateral menisci were excised, following placement of a Homén retractor to expose the proximal tibia. Anterior tibial osteophyte was resected. The tibial cut block was navigated into position and pinned in place. This was confirmed. The proximal tibial cut was made and verified. The 83 sizing plate was positioned and selected.

Extramedullary alignment was used to confirm alignment and was pinned in place. Stem punch was passed. Following this, the posterior cruciate ligament was excised, posterior condylar osteophytes were resected, and posterior capsular release was accomplished. The intercondylar notch guide was placed and the notch cut was made. With trials in place, the patient did require a subperiosteal medial release to balance the knee in both flexion and extension. The patella was resurfaced from 25 precut to 24 postcut using an inset patella with no-thumb tracking being quite excellent.

Answer Sheet

Directions: Be sure to enter all medical record codes in the manner provided in the sample below, paying special attention to the decimal placement for each code. The codes must be typed on the answer sheet in the boxes provided on the computer screen using the keyboard. A decimal point (.) has been provided as a guide for entering each ICD-9-CM code. **You will lose credit if the digits of the codes are correct, but the decimal point has been incorrectly placed.**

CASE 7 DIAGNOSES   **ICD-9-CM**

DX1				.		
DX2				.		
DX3				.		
DX4				.		

CASE 7 PROCEDURES   **CPT/HCPCS**

PR1					
PR2					
PR3					
PR4					
PR5					
PR6					

CASE STUDY 8

Please code for the services of the surgeon.

Practice Exam 2   CASE 8

ADMISSION DATE: 11/16/20XX

SURGERY DATE: 11/16/20XX

PREOPERATIVE DIAGNOSIS: Right renal calculi

POSTOPERATIVE DIAGNOSIS: Right renal calculi

PROCEDURE: Right percutaneous nephrolithotomy, placement of percutaneous nephrostomy tube, and placement of right double J ureteral stent, as well as nephroscopy.

SURGEON:

ASSISTANT: None

ESTIMATED BLOOD LOSS: 75 mL

SPECIMENS REMOVED: Multiple renal calculi

FINDINGS: Very hard renal calculus with satellite calculi requiring flexible nephroscopy, laser lithotripsy, as well as an upper pole calyceal diverticulum with a narrow neck

COMPLICATIONS: None

The patient is a 33-year-old man with significant history of nephrolithiasis. He is status post right sided pyeloplasty, as well as a prior percutaneous nephrolithotomy. He had a stone recurrence early in the year and wanted to wait to have this taken care of despite the risks of progressive renal damage. We reviewed the treatment options and he chose percutaneous nephrolithotomy despite the risks. These included, but are not limited to, bleeding, infection, renal damage, renal damage to the point of requiring dialysis or nephrectomy, bleeding requiring transfusion with associated risks such as HIV and hepatitis, MID, DVT, stroke, death, and pneumothorax. The patient understood and consented. On the date of the operation, a percutaneous access was obtained onto the ureter by interventional radiology. The patient was brought to the operating room and placed in supine position. General anesthesia was induced. He was then placed in the prone position and padded in the appropriate pressure points. The patient was then prepared and draped in the standard fashion. An implant guidewire was then placed down the patient's catheter into the bladder under fluoroscopic guidance. The tract was noted to be dense due to his prior surgery, but it was dilated up to 12-French sequentially with the implants dilators. A 2 wire introducer was then placed on the ureter and a second wire was placed into the patient's bladder. The nephroscopy dilating balloon was then placed under fluoroscopic guidance into the patient's renal pelvis. The balloon was insufflated to 18 atmospheres of pressure. The nephroscope sheath was placed over the balloon into the renal pelvis.

The balloon was desufflated and removed leaving a safety guidewire and a working guidewire. The stones were immediately identified. Using the ultrasonic laser lithotrite, a large satellite fragment was identified and attempted to be broken up. This ultrasonic laser lithotrite was used until it had actually broken. This was removed and we attempted to get another one while we incorporated the use of a laser fiber with a 500-micron fiber at settings of 1 joule and 10 Hz. The stone was then carefully lithotripped, so as to not create large fragments. Once the ultrasonic lithotrite was replaced, the laser was removed. The stone was then fragmented into large pieces. A number of pieces approximately 0.5 cm were then removed with grasping forceps. These were sent off the table as a specimen. Smaller specimens were then lithotripped until they were aspirated through the ultrasonic lithotrite. The nephroscope was removed. The flexible nephroscopy identified a large stone in the upper pole calyx. Of note, an additional stone was noted under fluoroscopic guidance in the upper pole and it was noted to be in a diverticulum with a small tract. The diverticulum was dilated with the flexible nephroscope. The stone was, however, intraparenchymal. During the course of this, the stone in the satellite calyx in the upper pole had fallen into the renal pelvis. The flexible nephroscope was removed and the rigid nephroscope was placed. The stone was crushed using the ultrasonic lithotrite and grasped and removed as well with the large grasping forceps. The collecting system was examined for small fragments and each one was grasped under fluoroscopic guidance. The entire kidney was noted to be cleaned of stones after the procedure. Using the guidewire, a double J 6-French × 26 cm stent was placed down the ureter into the bladder and noted to curl. It was then curled into the renal pelvis. A 10-French percutaneous nephroscopy tube was then placed in the renal pelvis into the upper pole, as to be away from the stent. The nephroscope sheath was removed. The percutaneous nephrostomy was locked into place and a nephrostogram was performed confirming the correct placement of both the double J ureteral stent and the percutaneous nephrostomy tube. The skin was then sutured closed using 2-0 silk and secured to the suture with the percutaneous nephrostomy tube. All tubes were then placed to gravity drainage. The patient was placed back in the supine position, awakened from anesthesia, and taken to the recovery room in stable condition.

Answer Sheet

Directions: Be sure to enter all medical record codes in the manner provided in the sample below, paying special attention to the decimal placement for each code. The codes must be typed on the answer sheet in the boxes provided on the computer screen using the keyboard. A decimal point (.) has been provided as a guide for entering each ICD-9-CM code. **You will lose credit if the digits of the codes are correct, but the decimal point has been incorrectly placed.**

CASE 8 DIAGNOSES   **ICD-9-CM**

DX1				.		
DX2				.		
DX3				.		
DX4				.		

CASE 8 PROCEDURES   **CPT/HCPCS**

PR1					
PR2					
PR3					
PR4					
PR5					
PR6					

CASE STUDY 9

Please code for the services of the surgeon.

Practice Exam 2   CASE 9

PREOPERATIVE DIAGNOSIS: Conn's syndrome with abnormal aldosterone secretion from the left adrenal gland

POSTOPERATIVE DIAGNOSIS: Conn's syndrome with abnormal aldosterone secretion from the left adrenal gland

OPERATION PERFORMED: Laparoscopic left adrenalectomy

ATTENDING SURGEON:

ANESTHESIA: General

ESTIMATED BLOOD LOSS: Less than 20 cc

FLUID REPLACEMENT: 1,000 cc lactated Ringer's solution

URINE OUTPUT: 175 cc

SPECIMENS: Left adrenal gland

INDICATIONS FOR PROCEDURE: This 46-year-old African-American woman has hypertension and hypokalemia. Her medications include Norvasc and potassium supplement. Workup revealed hyperaldosteronism that, after adrenal vein sampling, appeared to localize specifically to the left adrenal gland with markedly elevated levels of aldosterone. After the risks and benefits of the procedure and possible complications were explained, the patient elected to undergo laparoscopic left adrenalectomy.

DESCRIPTION OF PROCEDURE: The patient was brought to the operative suite and positioned on the operating room table in the right lateral decubitus position with the left side up. She was adequately padded and taped in position. She was then prepared and draped in the usual sterile fashion. Initial access to the abdomen was obtained using a direct cut-down technique below the left ribs. Insertion of a blunt cannula was undertaken and the abdomen was insufflated under direct visualization. There appeared to be limited working space in the abdomen due to the patient's central obesity and a large amount of intra-abdominal fat. In addition, the patient had a very large fatty liver that was clear over to the left abdomen. Under direct visualization, we placed a more medial 5.0-mm trocar in the left hypochondrium and in addition, two 5.0-mm trocars in the left hypochondrium more lateral to our initial access site.

We proceeded to mobilize the left colon from the left sidewall using harmonic shears and we adequately mobilized the colon out of the way. We then proceeded to roll the colon mesentery medially where we could identify Gerota's fascia.

We then followed Gerota's fascia superiorly and rolled the inferior pole of the spleen medially and superiorly, rolling the spleen off its left lateral attachments. This allowed us to identify the area of the adrenal gland. We then proceeded to open up Gerota's fascia gently using an L-hook cautery where we identified the adrenal gland in place, which appeared to be somewhat long and flat in appearance.

After completely opening up Gerota's fascia to expose the adrenal gland in its entirety, meticulous dissection was carried out inferiorly and medially where we identified a solitary left adrenal vein which we triply clipped and divided. Further L-hook cautery was then used to dissect the gland from the underlying fat. This was done with excellent hemostasis. Additional small blood vessels were clipped and divided and further dissection enabled identification of the left phrenic vein, which again was triply clipped and divided. We then further dissected the adrenal gland off its bed using L-hook cautery with excellent hemostasis. We then placed the gland into an impermeable entrapment sac and removed it through the initial access site, passing it off the field. Inspection of the adrenal bed revealed it to have good hemostasis. We irrigated with warm normal saline and aspirated back. There was no evidence of bleeding. We then proceeded to close our initial access trocar site with O Vicryl suture on a suture-passer using a figure-of-8 technique. The rest of the abdomen was inspected. We replaced the left colon back into the left upper abdomen. There was no injury to the colon throughout the entire procedure. The patient tolerated the procedure well.

We removed our instruments under direct visualization, desufflating the abdomen completely. There was no bleeding from the trocar sites. The patient's bed was unflexed and the fascial suture was tied. The skin and fascia were anesthetized with 0.25% Marcaine plain. The skin was closed with 4-0 monocryl subcuticular stitch. Steri-Strips were applied. Sterile dressing was applied. The patient was transferred to the recovery room in stable and satisfactory condition.

Answer Sheet

Directions: Be sure to enter all medical record codes in the manner provided in the sample below, paying special attention to the decimal placement for each code. The codes must be typed on the answer sheet in the boxes provided on the computer screen using the keyboard. A decimal point (.) has been provided as a guide for entering each ICD-9-CM code. **You will lose credit if the digits of the codes are correct, but the decimal point has been incorrectly placed.**

CASE 9 DIAGNOSES   **ICD-9-CM**

DX1				.		
DX2				.		
DX3				.		
DX4				.		

CASE 9 PROCEDURES   **CPT/HCPCS**

PR1					
PR2					
PR3					
PR4					
PR5					
PR6					

174

CASE STUDY 10

Please code for the services of the surgeon.

Practice Exam 2   CASE 10

PREOPERATIVE DIAGNOSIS: Ductal carcinoma in situ of the right breast

POSTOPERATIVE DIAGNOSIS: Ductal carcinoma in situ of the right breast

PROCEDURE:

1. Right needle-localized lumpectomy
2. Axillary sampling

ANESTHESIA: General endotracheal

ESTIMATED BLOOD LOSS: Minimal

FLUIDS: 1,000 cc

DISPOSITION: To recovery room

INDICATIONS: The patient is a 71-year-old woman who was noted to have abnormal calcifications at roughly the 6 o'clock position of the areola. These were biopsied and found to be ductal carcinoma in situ. She was inclined to proceed with needle-localized lumpectomy. The risks of bleeding, infection, poor wound healing, and unappealing cosmetics were discussed. The possibility we could find invasive carcinoma was also discussed. The need for postoperative radiation therapy was also discussed. She was well aware of the possibility of positive margins that would lead to further surgery or a mastectomy.

PROCEDURE: The patient was initially taken to the Center for Breast Diagnosis where Dr. X placed a needle at the inferior aspect of the breast.

The patient was then taken to the operating room. General anesthesia was administered. SCDs were placed. A curvilinear incision was made on the inferior aspect of the areola. This was taken down to the subcutaneous tissue. Flaps were raised in each direction for approximately 2 cm and taken down to the chest wall. A long stitch was placed medially, a short stitch superiorly.

The specimen was then removed. The cavity was then thoroughly irrigated. ¼% Marcaine was used for local anesthesia. A sampling of axillary lymph nodes were removed.

The subcutaneous tissue was then approximated using 3-0 Monocryl. The skin was approximated using 4-0 Monocryl in a running subcuticular fashion. A sterile dressing was then applied.

The patient tolerated the procedure well and was taken to the recovery room. The operative findings were discussed with her husband and daughter.

Answer Sheet

Directions: Be sure to enter all medical record codes in the manner provided in the sample below, paying special attention to the decimal placement for each code. The codes must be typed on the answer sheet in the boxes provided on the computer screen using the keyboard. A decimal point (.) has been provided as a guide for entering each ICD-9-CM code. **You will lose credit if the digits of the codes are correct, but the decimal point has been incorrectly placed.**

CASE 10 DIAGNOSES   **ICD-9-CM**

DX1				.		
DX2				.		
DX3				.		
DX4				.		

CASE 10 PROCEDURES   **CPT/HCPCS**

PR1					
PR2					
PR3					
PR4					
PR5					
PR6					

CASE STUDY 11

Please code for the services of the surgeon.

Practice Exam 2   CASE 11

DATE OF OPERATION: 10/26/20XX

PREOPERATIVE DIAGNOSIS: Hypertrophic pyloric stenosis

POSTOPERATIVE DIAGNOSES: Hypertrophic pyloric stenosis; thrombosed accessory spleen

OPERATION:

1. Laparoscopic pyloromyotomy
2. Excision of thrombosed accessory spleen

ANESTHESIA: General

INDICATIONS FOR SURGERY: Patient is a 4-week-old boy with a 1-week history of progressively projectile vomiting. Patient was brought to the emergency department where he underwent ultrasound evaluation. Ultrasound findings revealed a pyloric channel of 15 mm in length with a wall thickness of 3.8 mm, consistent with hypertrophic pyloric stenosis. Electrolytes were found to be within reasonable range. Patient is brought to the operating room for pyloromyotomy.

FINDINGS: Moderately hypertrophied pylorus. No evidence of mucosal perforation. There was a 1 cm × 2 cm dark purple mass on the omentum, consistent with a thrombosed accessory spleen. This was excised without difficulty and sent for pathologic evaluation.

PROCEDURE: After informed consent was obtained, the patient was brought to the operating suite and placed in supine position. After adequate endotracheal anesthesia had been administered, his stomach was decompressed and his bladder was emptied, and his abdomen was prepared and draped in the usual sterile fashion. After infiltration with a local anesthetic, the base of the umbilicus was everted and a vertical 5-mm incision was made. A Veress needle was introduced and pneumoperitoneum was established to 8 mm Hg pressure at 1 L/minute flow. The Veress needle was then replaced with a radially expandible 5-mm trocar. Laparascope was introduced and confirmed good placement. Under laparoscopic visualization, stab incisions were made in the right upper quadrant and left upper quadrant. In the right upper quadrant, a pyloric grasper was introduced and in the left upper quadrant, the Arthro blade was introduced. Examination revealed a 1 cm × 2 cm dark purplish mass attached to the omentum near the spleen. This was separate from the spleen. He had a normal appearing lobulated spleen in the left upper quadrant. This mass was consistent with a thrombosed accessory spleen. Following the stomach distally, the pyloric channel was identified. This was moderately hypertrophied, consistent with the ultrasound diagnosis. While the pylorus was stabilized, the Arthro blade was extruded approximately 2 mm and used to incise the pylorus. The blade was then retracted and the blunt tip was used to initiate the pyloromyotomy.

This then was replaced with a pyloric spreader, which was used to complete the pyloromyotomy. The mucosa was seen bulging without evidence of mucosal perforation. The pyloromyotomy was extended onto the antrum of the stomach. After there was good bulge of the mucosa, and the superior and inferior edges of the cut pylorus were independently mobile, the duodenum was occluded, and 40 cc of air was inflated into the stomach by the anesthesiologist. This revealed no evidence of a mucosal perforation. The stomach was then decompressed.

The laparoscope was removed and a 5-mm trocar was placed in the right upper quadrant incision site. Laparoscope confirmed good placement. The umbilical trocar was removed and the umbilical incision was slightly extended to allow placement of an Endo catch bag. Prior to the introduction of the Endo catch bag, the lesion on the omentum was dissected free using electrocautery. There was good hemostasis. The Endo catch bag was then introduced through the umbilical trocar site and was used to retrieve the lesion without spillage or contamination. On palpation, this was soft but solid, consistent with a thrombosed accessory spleen. This was sent for pathologic review.

Reexamination of the intraperitoneal cavity revealed good hemostasis. All instruments and trocars were removed and the pneumoperitoneum was deflated. The fascia of the right upper quadrant trocar site and the umbilical trocar site were closed with 2-0 Vicryl in figure-of-8 stitch fashion. The umbilical skin incision was closed with 5-0 plain gut in interrupted stitch fashion. The other upper quadrant incisions were closed with Monocryl in subcuticular running stitch fashion. All incisions were cleaned and infiltrated with a local anesthetic. The umbilical trocar site was dressed with sterile gauze and Tegaderm. The other incisions were dressed with Steri-Strips. The patient tolerated the procedure well, was extubated, and then returned to the recovery room in stable condition.

Pathology Report

CLINICAL INFORMATION

PROCEDURE: Laparoscopic pyloromyotomy

PREOPERATIVE DIAGNOSIS: Pyloric stenosis (thrombosed accessory spleen)

CLINICAL HISTORY: Not given

GROSS DESCRIPTION:
Received fresh for routine examination designated R/O ACCESSORY SPLEEN is a 0.6 g, 1.1 cm × 1.0 cm × 0.5 cm, red-brown nodule with external smooth, glistening surface. The specimen is bisected and submitted entirely in one cassette.

MICROSCOPIC DESCRIPTION:
Sections through the accessory spleen revealed subcapsular markedly congested splenic sinusoids with minimal periarteriolar lymphocytic aggregates. Centrally the splenic tissue displays marked congestion and hemorrhage with loss of the sinusoidal pattern. Instead the parenchyma is largely replaced by capillaries with an intervening loose fibrin meshwork. At the periphery the hilum of the accessory spleen contains an extensive neutrophilic infiltrate. Scattered calcified nodules are noted within the splenic parenchyma.

DIAGNOSIS:
ABDOMINAL NODULE, EXCISION: ACCESSORY SPLEEN WITH CONGESTION AND HEMORRHAGE

Answer Sheet

Directions: Be sure to enter all medical record codes in the manner provided in the sample below, paying special attention to the decimal placement for each code. The codes must be typed on the answer sheet in the boxes provided on the computer screen using the keyboard. A decimal point (.) has been provided as a guide for entering each ICD-9-CM code. **You will lose credit if the digits of the codes are correct, but the decimal point has been incorrectly placed.**

CASE 11 DIAGNOSES   **ICD-9-CM**

DX1				.		
DX2				.		
DX3				.		
DX4				.		

CASE 11 PROCEDURES   **CPT/HCPCS**

PR1					
PR2					
PR3					
PR4					
PR5					
PR6					

CASE STUDY 12

Please code for the services of the surgeon.

Practice Exam 2   CASE 12

DATE OF OPERATION: 09/25/20XX

PREOPERATIVE DIAGNOSES:

1. Left facial skin tag
2. Left preauricular sinus

POSTOPERATIVE DIAGNOSES:

1. Left facial skin tag
2. Left preauricular sinus

OPERATION:

1. Excision of left facial skin tag
2. Excision of left preauricular sinus tract with wound closure 1.1 cm

ANESTHESIA: General endotracheal anesthesia

FLUIDS: Approximately 100 cc crystalloid

ESTIMATED BLOOD LOSS: Less than 5 cc

URINE OUTPUT: None

CULTURES: None

DRAINS: None

SPECIMENS:

1. Left facial skin tag
2. Left preauricular sinus

FINDINGS: 1.1 cm left preauricular sinus and approximately 1 cm left facial skin tag

DESCRIPTION OF PROCEDURE: The patient was brought to the operating room. General endotracheal anesthesia was introduced. The table was turned 90° counterclockwise. The skin and subcutaneous tissue around the sinus as well as the left facial skin tag were infiltrated with 0.5% Marcaine with 1:100,000 epinephrine. A total of 1.5 cc was used. The patient was then prepared and draped in the usual sterile fashion.

Attention was first turned to the sinus and a lacrimal probe was used to determine the extent and direction of the sinus. The tract was approximately 1.1 cm and the outline was made with a marking pen followed by incision through the skin and dermis with a Weck blade. Sharpie scissors were then used to dissect down to the sinus capsule and dissect out the capsule until it was removed and blocked. Hemostasis was then achieved and the wound was closed in 3 layers; 1 to obliterate the subcutaneous tissues with 4-0 Vicryl simple interrupted followed by a single deep dermal of 4-0 Vicryl and finally the skin was reapproximated with a 6-0 fast absorbing gut running subcuticular suture.

Attention was then turned to the skin tag and it was removed with a single snip of tenotomy scissors. The resulting wound was then reapproximated with a single 6-0 fast absorbing gut simple interrupted suture. The wound was dressed with Tegaderm and care of the patient returned to the anesthesia team.

COMPLICATIONS: None

DISPOSITION: To the postanesthesia care unit

Pathology Report

CLINICAL INFORMATION

PROCEDURE: Excision of left preauricular skin tag and sinus

PREOPERATIVE DIAGNOSIS: Preauricular skin tag and sinus, left

CLINICAL HISTORY: None given

GROSS DESCRIPTION:

1. Received in formalin for routine examination designated LEFT PREAURICULAR SINUS is a tan irregular fragment of tissue measuring $0.8 \times 0.3 \times 0.2$ cm. The entire specimen is submitted in cassette A.

2. Received in formalin for routine examination designated SKIN TAG, LEFT PRE-AURICULAR is a cone-shaped fragment of tissue lined by skin measuring 0.5 cm in length with a variable diameter from 0.2 cm at the base to 0.1 cm at the tip. The cut margin is inked black. The specimen is bisected, wrapped, and submitted in cassette B.

MICROSCOPIC DESCRIPTION:

1. Microscopic sections examined; description omitted.

2. The facial skin tag is covered by keratinizing squamous epithelium with underlying intact adenxal structures and a central core of skeletal muscle.

DIAGNOSIS:

1. LEFT PREAURICULAR SINUS, EXCISION: DERMOID SINUS

2. LEFT PREAURICULAR SKIN TAG, EXCISION: HARMATOMATOUS MALFORMATION OF SKIN AND SKELETAL MUSCLE. SEE COMMENT

COMMENT:

Although the pathology requisition identifies the resected skin tag as coming from the left preauricular region, the clinic note from 8/24/20XX instead indicates that this skin tag was located posterolateral to the lateral canthus of the left eye.

Answer Sheet

Directions: Be sure to enter all medical record codes in the manner provided in the sample below, paying special attention to the decimal placement for each code. The codes must be typed on the answer sheet in the boxes provided on the computer screen using the keyboard. A decimal point (.) has been provided as a guide for entering each ICD-9-CM code. **You will lose credit if the digits of the codes are correct, but the decimal point has been incorrectly placed.**

CASE 12 DIAGNOSES   **ICD-9-CM**

DX1				.		
DX2				.		
DX3				.		
DX4				.		

CASE 12 PROCEDURES   **CPT/HCPCS**

PR1					
PR2					
PR3					
PR4					
PR5					
PR6					

CASE STUDY 13

Please code for the services of the surgeon.

Practice Exam 2 CASE 13

PREOPERATIVE DIAGNOSIS: Intraocular foreign body

POSTOPERATIVE DIAGNOSIS: Intraocular foreign body

PROCEDURE: Pars plana vitrectomy. Removal of intraocular foreign body.

ANESTHESIA: General endotracheal tube

PROCEDURE IN DETAIL: After induction of general anesthesia the patient was prepared and draped in a sterile fashion and a lid speculum placed. Monitoring of intraocular pressure was begun and maintained throughout the procedure. A free port pars plana vitrectomy was initiated and anterior vitrectomy of the anterior vitreous was done. This was followed by examination of the posterior pole. The view was significantly obstructed due to a significant corneal scar through the center of the cornea. We cautiously cleaned the vitreous until we were confident that the retina was not detached and we did a 360° removal of the posterior hyaloid and a very opaque vitreous. We identified an intraocular foreign body that was nonmetallic because it did not rise when we used the intraocular magnet. After this we placed some Perfluoron to protect the macular area although there was some swelling of the macula and a small hemorrhage of the retina in the macular area but it did not appear that any retinal hole, tear, or detachment was present. We grabbed the foreign body with forceps because of its very large size and did approximately a 5-mm wound extending from the temporal sclerotomy in order to remove the large intraocular foreign body. After the foreign body was removed we removed the remaining Perfluoron, examined the peripheral retina, and we did not see obvious tears or detachments. After this, we closed the sclerotomy wounds with 8-0 nylon suture and the conjunctiva with an 8-0 Vicryl suture. After this, we did a subtenon block of anesthesia for comfort and following this we used a little Tisseel glue on the surface of the cornea and put a bandage contact lens as from previous repair the patient had had corneal glue on the eye that was very rough and uncomfortable. Following this, the eye was patched and shielded with a sterile patch and some Maxitrol ointment was applied to the eye. There were no complications. Specimens sent to pathology. There were no drains or packs. Our plan is to admit the patient overnight and will follow the patient tomorrow.

Answer Sheet

Directions: Be sure to enter all medical record codes in the manner provided in the sample below, paying special attention to the decimal placement for each code. The codes must be typed on the answer sheet in the boxes provided on the computer screen using the keyboard. A decimal point (.) has been provided as a guide for entering each ICD-9-CM code. **You will lose credit if the digits of the codes are correct, but the decimal point has been incorrectly placed.**

CASE 13 DIAGNOSES   **ICD-9-CM**

					.		
DX1					.		
DX2					.		
DX3					.		
DX4					.		

CASE 13 PROCEDURES   **CPT/HCPCS**

PR1					
PR2					
PR3					
PR4					
PR5					
PR6					

CASE STUDY 14

Please code for the services of the physician.

Practice Exam 2   CASE 14

NEW PATIENT

CHIEF COMPLAINT: Cough

HISTORY OF PRESENT ILLNESS: The patient is a 64-year-old woman who presents to my office with 1 week of cough. She has initially had small amounts of a whitish-type sputum that was productive, but this has resolved and now her cough is productive only occasionally of clear sputum. She has had no fevers or chills. Her cough, however, is unrelenting and somewhat paroxysmal to the point where she is unable to sleep. She has chest discomfort only with cough and not with inspiratory effort, and there is no exertional worsening of her chest discomfort. She is not particularly short of breath, other than that which is produced by her paroxysms of coughing.

PAST MEDICAL HISTORY:

1. Hypertension
2. Rheumatoid arthritis
3. Type II diabetes

There is no history of ischemic heart disease.

PAST SURGICAL HISTORY: The patient is status post left knee replacement, 15 years ago.

CURRENT MEDICATIONS:

1. Avandia
2. HCTZ
3. Azathioprine
4. Methotrexate
5. Prempro
6. Metformin
7. Enalapril
8. Azithromycin, day #3
9. Elavil
10. Remicade

ALLERGIES: No known drug allergies.

SOCIAL HISTORY: The patient lives independently with her husband. She drinks minimal ethanol. Does not use tobacco.

FAMILY HISTORY: Negative

REVIEW OF SYSTEMS:

GENERAL: No recent fevers or chills. Appetite has been intact.

ENT: No upper respiratory symptoms or sore throat

NECK: No neck pain or stiffness

PULMONARY: See history of present illness.

CARDIOVASCULAR: See history of present illness.

GASTROINTESTINAL: No abdominal pain, vomiting, or stool changes

PHYSICAL EXAMINATION:

VITAL SIGNS: Blood pressure is 182/86. Pulse is 109. Respirations 22. Temperature is 99.8 degrees. O_2 saturation on room air 98%.

GENERAL: The patient is awake and alert. She has paroxysms of coughing and is uncomfortable, but otherwise is nontoxic.

HEENT: Sclerae are anicteric. Palpebral conjunctivae are pink. TMs are clear bilaterally. There is no purulent nasal discharge or sinus tenderness. The oropharynx is clear. Neck is supple. No JVD or bruits noted.

LUNGS: Breath sounds are somewhat diminished at the bases, but are clear. There is no prolongation of the expiratory phase or other evidence of respiratory distress, other than this paroxysmal cough.

CARDIAC: Regular, S1 and S2. No murmur or gallop appreciated.

ABDOMEN: Soft, nontender, without hepatosplenomegaly or mass

EXTREMITIES: No clubbing edema. There are deformities consistent with the patient's known history of rheumatoid arthritis. Pulses are full and symmetric throughout.

SKIN: Warm and dry. No jaundice, pallor, or cyanosis noted.

NEUROLOGIC: The patient is alert, fully oriented. Pupils equal, round, reactive to light. The remainder of her examination is nonfocal.

An albuterol 2.5 mg and atrovent 0.5 mg nebulizer treatment was given ×1 as a diagnostic therapeutic trial. The patient's posttreatment peak flows were 200, but her aeration was increased and her cough was noticeably lessened. She was sent to the radiology suite for a chest x-ray, PA and lateral. This revealed no acute infiltrates or other acute pulmonary disease. Blood pressure has been elevated and is being monitored 3 times per day. Glucose levels are monitored in the morning and the evening. My findings and recommendations were subsequently discussed with the patient and her husband in detail. I have recommended she continue her current medications, including the azithromycin prescribed by her physician. Combivent 2 puffs q.4 h. p.r.n. with a spacer was prescribed for cough and apparent bronchospasm. MDI teaching was performed by respiratory therapy and the patient was given a spacer for her use. Tessalon Perles, 1-2 q.6 h. p.r.n. was also given to her for additional cough relief. She should follow up with me in 2 to 3 days.

DIAGNOSES:

Acute bronchitis
Hypertension
Rheumatoid arthritis
Diabetes, type II

HISTORY: Detailed

EXAMINATION: Comprehensive

MEDICAL DECISION-MAKING: Moderate

Answer Sheet

Directions: Be sure to enter all medical record codes in the manner provided in the sample below, paying special attention to the decimal placement for each code. The codes must be typed on the answer sheet in the boxes provided on the computer screen using the keyboard. A decimal point (.) has been provided as a guide for entering each ICD-9-CM code. **You will lose credit if the digits of the codes are correct, but the decimal point has been incorrectly placed.**

CASE 14 DIAGNOSES   ICD-9-CM

DX1				.		
DX2				.		
DX3				.		
DX4				.		

CASE 14 PROCEDURES   CPT/HCPCS

PR1					
PR2					
PR3					
PR4					
PR5					
PR6					

CASE STUDY 15

Please code for the services of the physician.

Practice Exam 2   CASE 15

DIAGNOSIS: s/p Tetralogy of Fallot repair

INDICATIONS: Palpitations

A two-channel Holter monitor was recorded for 23:59 hours. The predominant rhythm was sinus rhythm with sinus arrhythmia and wandering atrial pacemaker. Analysis of the recording revealed that the heart rate ranged from 70 to 145 bpm with an average heart rate of 99 bpm.

Supraventricular arrhythmias occurred. The mean frequency of supraventricular premature depolarizations was 0.7 beats per hour. The frequency ranged from 0 to 6 for a total of 16 beats. This represents < .01% of the rhythm.

Supraventricular tachycardia occurred. 1 episode(s) occurred. The longest run was 3 beats. The fastest run was 118 bpm.

Ventricular arrhythmia did not occur. Ventricular couplets did not occur. Ventricular tachycardia did not occur. AV block did not occur. Bradycardia for patient's age was not recorded.

ECG Intervals: PR = 120–160 msec   QRS = 120 msec   QTc = 436–481 msec

No symptoms were recorded during the monitoring period.

IMPRESSION:

The quality of the tracing was good.

1. The predominant rhythm was normal sinus rhythm with sinus arrhythmia and wandering atrial pacemaker. Physiologic and circadian heart rate variation were mildly diminished. The heart rate ranged from 70 to 145 bpm, averaging 99 bpm.

2. Rare supraventricular premature beats occurred, comprising < 0.01% of the total rhythm. There was 1 supraventricular couplet with a coupling interval of 0.560 msec.

3. Ventricular ectopy will not occur. Neither ventricular couplets nor runs occurred. VT did not occur.

4. Bradycardia did not occur. AV block did not occur.

5. No definite diagnosis identified.

Answer Sheet

Directions: Be sure to enter all medical record codes in the manner provided in the sample below, paying special attention to the decimal placement for each code. The codes must be typed on the answer sheet in the boxes provided on the computer screen using the keyboard. A decimal point (.) has been provided as a guide for entering each ICD-9-CM code. **You will lose credit if the digits of the codes are correct, but the decimal point has been incorrectly placed.**

CASE 15 DIAGNOSES ICD-9-CM

				.		
DX1				.		
DX2				.		
DX3				.		
DX4				.		

CASE 15 PROCEDURES CPT/HCPCS

PR1					
PR2					
PR3					
PR4					
PR5					
PR6					

CASE STUDY 16

Please code for the services of the laboratory.

Practice Exam 2   CASE 16

Laboratory Results

CLINICAL HISTORY: Hyperemesis gravidarum with electrolyte imbalance at 21 weeks gestation

Drawn here today.

03/10/20XX 13:00 Basic Metabolic Panel			For more Final Results Received	
Specimen Comment	1 SERUM SEPARATOR TUBE (SST)			Final
Sodium	137		[136–145 mmol/L]	Final
Potassium	3.3	L	[3.8–5.4 mmol/L]	Final
Chloride	95	L	[98–106 mmol/L]	Final
Carbon Dioxide	36	H	[20–26 mmol/L]	Final
BUN	14		[7–18 mg/dL]	Final
Creatinine	0.8		[0.4–1.0 md/dL]	Final
Glucose	114	H	[70–106 mg/dL]	Final
Calcium (total)	7.7	L	[8.8–10.1 mg/dL]	Final

03/10/20XX 13:00 CBC with Auto Diff			For more Final Results Received	
White Blood Cell Count	10.8		[4.5–13.5 THOU/uL]	Final
Red Blood Cell Count	3.56	L	[4.5–5.3 MIL/uL]	Final
Hemoglobin	10.8	L	[13.0–16.0 g/dL]	Final
Hematocrit	31.3	L	[37.0–49.0 %]	Final
Mean Corpuscular Volume	87.8		[78.0–98.0 fL]	Final
Mean Corpuscular Hgb	30.4		[25.0–35.0 pg]	Final
Mean Corpus Hgb Conc	34.5		[31.0–37.0 g/dL]	Final
Red Distribution Width	15.7	H	[11.5–14.5 %]	Final
Platelet Count	95	LL	[150–400 THOU/uL]	Final
CONSISTENT WITH PREVIOUS RESULTS				
Mean Platelet Volume	7.3	L	[7.4–10.4 fL]	Final
Segmented Neutrophils	95.7	H	[40–59 %]	Final
Absolute Neutrophil Count	10336		[THOU/uL]	Final
Eosinophils Count	0.6		[0–4 %]	Final
Basophils	0		[0–1 %]	Final
Lymphocytes	1.4	L	[34–48 %]	Final
Monocytes	2.3	L	[3–8 %]	Final
Platelet Estimate	Not Done			Final
Differential Method	AUTOMATED			Final

Answer Sheet

Directions: Be sure to enter all medical record codes in the manner provided in the sample below, paying special attention to the decimal placement for each code. The codes must be typed on the answer sheet in the boxes provided on the computer screen using the keyboard. A decimal point (.) has been provided as a guide for entering each ICD-9-CM code. **You will lose credit if the digits of the codes are correct, but the decimal point has been incorrectly placed.**

CASE 16 DIAGNOSES   **ICD-9-CM**

DX1					.		
DX2					.		
DX3					.		
DX4					.		

CASE 16 PROCEDURES   **CPT/HCPCS**

PR1					
PR2					
PR3					
PR4					
PR5					
PR6					

Practice Exam 3
Multiple Choice Questions

Domain 1: Health Information Documentation

1. Which reference book would be used by the coder to determine which diagnosis from the problem list is treated by a drug prescribed by the physician?

    a. *Taber's Cyclopedic Medical Dictionary*

    b. *Gray's Anatomy*

    c. *Physicians' Desk Reference*

    d. *Medicine—Current Clinical Strategies*

2. What is the name of the formal document prepared by a surgeon at the conclusion of surgery to describe the surgical procedure performed?

    a. Operative report

    b. Tissue report

    c. Pathology report

    d. Anesthesia record

3. On what form would the following be documented, "Chest x-ray, AP and Lateral, to rule out pneumonia"?

    a. Progress notes

    b. Physical examination

    c. Physician's orders

    d. Nursing notes

4. All of the following information is needed to correctly code skin grafts except:

    a. Size of the defect

    b. Location of the donor site

    c. Type of graft used

    d. Location of the defect

5. What information is needed to correctly assign a CPT Emergency Department code?

    a. Whether the patient is new or established to the emergency department physician

    b. How much time the physician spent with the patient

    c. What was the level of history, examination, and medical decision-making

    d. Whether the physician is an employee of the hospital

6. A coder has a question about how to use a newly created ICD-9-CM code. What would be the best reference?

    a. *CPT Assistant*

    b. *Coding Clinic*

    c. Local coverage determinations (LCDs)

    d. Correct coding initiatives

Domain 2: ICD-9-CM Diagnosis Coding

7. In ICD-9-CM, the name of a disease, structure, operation, or procedure, usually derived from the name of the person who discovered or described it first is known as a(n):

    a. Carryover line

    b. Nonessential modifier

    c. Inclusion note

    d. Eponym

8. The symbol in ICD-9-CM's Tabular List used after an incomplete term that needs one or more of the modifiers that follows so that it can be assigned to a given category or code is:

    a. Colon

    b. Section mark

    c. Brace

    d. Lozenge

9. This symbol in ICD-9-CM encloses supplementary words or explanatory information that may or may not be present in the statement of a diagnosis or procedure:

    a. Square brackets

    b. Colon

    c. Parentheses

    d. Brace

10. A symptom, as defined in ICD-9-CM, is the:

    a. Condition established after study to be responsible for a patient's admission to hospital

    b. Subjective evidence of disease reported by the patient to the physician

    c. Objective evidence of a disease as observed by a physician

    d. Type of procedure performed for definite treatment of a patient

11. When coding sepsis and severe sepsis, which code should be sequenced first?

    a. Code for the postprocedural infection

    b. Code from subcategory 995.9 (SIRS)

    c. Code for the associated organ dysfunction(s)

    d. Code for the systemic infection

12. This elderly female patient was seen today in the physician's office for the administration of her first radiation treatment for glioblastoma multiforme, which was recently diagnosed. The diagnosis was listed as: Radiotherapy for management of glioblastoma multiforme in her right occipital lobe.

V58.0	Encounter for radiotherapy
V58.11	Encounter for antineoplastic chemotherapy
V58.12	Encounter for antineoplastic immunotherapy
191.4	Malignant neoplasm of brain, occipital lobe
191.6	Malignant neoplasm of brain, cerebellum, NOS
191.9	Malignant neoplasm of brain, unspecified

    a. V58.0; 191.4

    b. V58.12; 191.6

    c. V58.0; 191.9

    d. V58.11; 191.4

13. A 55-year-old morbidly obese woman with familial hypercholesterolemia was seen in her physician's office for a follow-up visit. She has managed to control her condition with medication and was also counseled at this time to maintain her smoke-free status. An appointment was set up for a return visit in four months.

272.0	Pure hypercholesterolemia
272.4	Other and unspecified hyperlipidemia
278.00	Obesity, unspecified
278.01	Morbid obesity
278.02	Overweight

    a. 272.0; 278.00

    b. 272.4; 278.02

    c. 272.0; 278.01

    d. 272.4; 278.00

14. The patient with paranoid alcoholic psychosis is seen in the physician's office for a follow-up visit. Upon questioning, the patient reluctantly admits to experiencing some delusions and to an intake of large amounts of alcohol on a continuous basis. The physician schedules another appointment for the patient in one month.

> 291.3 Alcohol-induced psychotic disorder with hallucinations
>
> 291.4 Idiosyncratic alcohol intoxication
>
> 291.5 Alcohol-induced psychotic disorder with delusions
>
> 303.0 Acute alcoholic intoxication
>
> 303.9 Other and unspecified alcohol dependence
>
> Fifth digits for use with Category 303:
>
>   0 unspecified
>
>   1 continuous
>
>   2 episodic
>
>   3 in remission

   a. 291.3; 303.00

   b. 291.5; 303.91

   c. 291.4; 303.01

   d. 291.5; 303.92

15. A 65-year-old woman was seen in the ophthalmologist's office for an annual eye examination. The patient was known to have chronic narrow-angle glaucoma in her right eye so the physician has been diligent in checking her left eye for glaucoma also. It was noted that the intraocular pressure in the left eye was now quite high as well, resulting in a diagnosis of acute narrow-angle glaucoma in that eye.

> 365.20 Primary angle-closure glaucoma, unspecified
>
> 365.21 Intermittent angle-closure glaucoma
>
> 365.22 Acute angle-closure glaucoma
>
> 365.23 Chronic angle-closure glaucoma
>
> 365.24 Residual stage of angle-closure glaucoma

   a. 365.22, 365.23

   b. 365.20; 365.21

   c. 365.24; 365.20

   d. 365.22; 365.21

16. An 84-year-old woman is seen in the hematologist's office for pernicious anemia that has been recently diagnosed. This patient is also known to have agammaglobulinemia, a frequent occurrence in patients with pernicious anemia. This patient is also being treated for chronic atrophic gastritis, another condition associated with her anemia. She is being treated with medications for these conditions and will return to the hematologist's office in two months.

> 279.00 Hypogammaglobulinemia, unspecified
>
> 279.06 Hypogammaglobulinemia, acquired
>
> 281.0   Pernicious anemia
>
> 281.8   Anemia associated with other specified nutritional deficiency
>
> 281.9   Unspecified deficiency anemia
>
> 535.10 Atrophic gastritis, without hemorrhage
>
> 535.11 Atrophic gastritis, with hemorrhage
>
> 535.00 Acute gastritis, without hemorrhage
>
> 535.40 Other specified gastritis without mention of hemorrhage

    a. 281.9; 279.06; 535.11

    b. 281.0; 279.06; 535.10

    c. 281.9; 279.06; 535.4

    d. 281.8; 279.00; 535.00

17. The patient is a 79-year-old man who is being seen in the physician's office for follow-up of his condition and medication renewals. This patient has congestive heart failure resulting from his malignant hypertension, chronic kidney disease, stage III, and type II diabetes with polyneuropathy. The patient has been a diabetic for many years.

> 404.01 Malignant hypertensive heart disease with heart failure and with chronic kidney disease stage I through stage IV, or unspecified
>
> 404.11 Benign hypertensive heart disease with heart failure and with chronic kidney disease stage I through stage IV, or unspecified
>
> 404.93 Unspecified hypertensive heart disease with heart failure and chronic kidney disease stage V or end stage renal disease
>
> 428.0   Unspecified congestive heart failure
>
> 429.9   Unspecified heart disease
>
> 585.2   Chronic kidney disease, stage II
>
> 585.3   Chronic kidney disease, stage III
>
> 250.60 Diabetes (type II or unspecified type) with neurological manifestations
>
> 250.61 Diabetes (type I [juvenile type]) with neurological manifestations
>
> 250.70 Diabetes (type II or unspecified type) with peripheral circulatory disorders
>
> 357.2   Polyneuropathy in diabetes
>
> 357.4   Polyneuropathy in other diseases classified elsewhere

    a. 404.01; 428.0; 585.3; 250.60; 357.2

    b. 404.93; 428.0; 585.2; 250.70; 357.4

    c. 404.11; 429.9; 585.3; 250.61; 357.4

    d. 404.01; 429.9; 585.2; 250.70; 357.2

18. A 12-year-old girl comes to the physician's office with her grandmother because of the following complaints: fever, discolored nasal discharge, puffy eyes, stuffy nose, and pain in the cheek areas. She was checked by the physician who confirmed all of her complaints and also detected fluid in her sinuses. The physician diagnosed acute sinusitis in the maxillary and frontal sinuses and prescribed antibiotics and Tylenol.

461.0	Acute maxillary sinusitis
461.1	Acute frontal sinusitis
461.8	Other acute sinusitis
461.9	Unspecified acute sinusitis
473.0	Chronic maxillary sinusitis
473.1	Chronic frontal sinusitis
473.9	Unspecified chronic sinusitis

   a. 473.0; 461.8

   b. 461.9; 473.9

   c. 461.8; 473.0

   d. 461.0, 461.1

19. The patient is a 57-year-old man who comes to the emergency department with severe abdominal pain. An acute gastric ulcer was identified following testing. There was no sign of malignancy or bleeding. The patient was placed on a special diet and discharged home.

   a. 531.70: Chronic gastric ulcer without mention of hemorrhage or perforation and without obstruction

   b. 531.30: Acute gastric ulcer without mention of hemorrhage or perforation and without obstruction

   c. 531.71: Chronic gastric ulcer without mention of hemorrhage or perforation and with obstruction

   d. 531.31: Acute gastric ulcer without mention of hemorrhage or perforation and with obstruction

20. This patient is seen for a follow-up visit because of a possible urinary tract infection. The patient was initially seen in the office about two days ago with complaints of urinating frequently, abdominal pressure, and burning on urination. A urinalysis was done, resulting in a diagnosis of acute cystitis due to *Escherichia coli* organism.

041.2	Bacterial infection in conditions classified elsewhere, and of unspecified site, *Pneumococcus*
041.4	Bacterial infection in conditions classified elsewhere, and of unspecified site, *Escherichia coli*
041.7	Bacterial infection in conditions classified elsewhere, and of unspecified site, *Pseudomonas*
595.0	Acute cystitis
595.1	Chronic interstitial cystitis
595.4	Cystitis in diseases classified elsewhere

   a. 595.0; 041.4

   b. 595.1; 041.2

   c. 595.4; 041.4

   d. 595.0; 041.7

Domain 3: CPT and HCPCS II Coding

21. The excised diameter of a lesion means the measurement of:

   a. The largest lesion dimension

   b. The largest lesion dimension and the measurement of the margin

   c. The largest lesion dimension and the measurement of both margins

   d. Both lesion dimensions added together and the measurement of the margin

22. The patient presents to the physician's office with fever and chills and is diagnosed with pneumonia. The physician administers 600 mg of Rocephin, IV over 1 hour and 31 minutes. In addition to the E/M code, how are these services coded?

J0696	Injection, Ceftriaxone sodium (Rocephin), per 250 mg
96365	Intravenous infusion, for therapy, prophylaxis, or diagnosis (specify substance or drug); initial, up to 1 hour
96366	each additional hour (List separately in addition to code for primary procedure)
96374	Therapeutic, prophylactic or diagnostic injection (specify substance or drug); intravenous push, single or initial substance/drug

   a. 96374, J0696

   b. 96365, J0696 × 2

   c. 96365, 96366, J0696

   d. 96365, 96366, J0696 × 3

23. In which HCPCS category would the coder find temporary codes for screening cyto-pathology to code services provided to patients covered by Medicare?

    a. G0008–G9143

    b. J0120–J9999

    c. K0001–K0899

    d. Q0035–Q9968

24. A 67-year-old patient is treated in the office today for a 5.0 cm × 3.0 cm full-thickness venous stasis ulcer of the lower leg. It was débrided previously. A skin graft of Apligraf, a tissue-cultured allogeneic skin substitute, is placed in the entire wound and is sutured in place. How would these physician services be coded?

15330	Acellular dermal allograft, trunk, arms, legs; first 100 sq cm or less, or 1% of body area of infants and children
15340	Tissue-cultured allogeneic skin substitute; first 25 sq cm or less
15360	Tissue-cultured allogeneic dermal substitute, trunk, arms, legs; first 100 sq cm or less, or 1% of body area of infants and children
Q4100	Skin substitute, not otherwise specified
Q4101	Skin substitute, apligraf, per square centimeter

    a. 15330, Q4100 ×5

    b. 15340, Q4100

    c. 15340, Q4101 ×15

    d. 15360, Q4101 ×8

25. When should the coder assign a code for a cast application?

    a. When applying a removable splint

    b. When revising a cast the patient is now wearing

    c. When a fracture treatment has been provided

    d. When applying a replacement cast during or after the period of normal follow-up care

26. The patient undergoes a left heart catheterization and a left ventricular angiography using percutaneous femoral access. How is this procedure coded?

93510	Left heart catheterization, retrograde, from the brachial artery, axillary artery or femoral artery; percutaneous
93514	Left heart catheterization by left ventricular puncture
93524	Combined transseptal and retrograde left heart catheterization
93543	Injection procedure during cardiac catheterization; for selective left ventricular or left atrial angiography
93544	for aortography
93555	Imaging supervision, interpretation and report for injection procedure(s) during cardiac catheterization; ventricular and/or atrial angiography
93556	pulmonary angiography, aortography, and/or selective coronary angiography including venous bypass grafts and arterial conduits (whether native or used in bypass)

a. 93510, 93543, 93555

b. 93510, 93544, 93556

c. 93514, 93544

d. 93524, 93543, 93556

27. The patient undergoes an arthroscopic débridement of the articular cartilage and removal of meniscus in the lateral compartment of the right knee. How is this procedure coded?

29870	Arthroscopy, knee, diagnostic, with or without synovial biopsy (separate procedure)
29877	Arthroscopy, knee, surgical; débridement/shaving of articular cartilage (chondroplasty)
29881	with meniscectomy (medial OR lateral, including any meniscal shaving)
29882	with meniscus repair (medial OR lateral)

a. 29881

b. 29877, 29881

c. 29877, 29882

d. 29870, 29877, 29881

28. The patient undergoes a proctosigmoidoscopy, a sigmoidoscopy with biopsy, and a colonoscopy during the same operative session. What is the correct coding assignment for these services?

45300	Proctosigmoidoscopy, rigid; diagnostic, with or without collection of specimen(s) by brushing or washing (separate procedure)
45305	with biopsy, single or multiple
45330	Sigmoidoscopy, flexible; diagnostic, with or without collection of specimen(s) by brushing or washing (separate procedure)
45331	with biopsy, single or multiple
45378	Colonoscopy, flexible, proximal to splenic flexure; diagnostic, with or without collection of specimen(s) by brushing or washing, with or without colon decompression (separate procedure)
45380	with biopsy, single or multiple

a. 45378

b. 45380

c. 45300, 45331, 45378

d. 45305, 45331, 45380

29. A physician's office performs an x-ray. The radiologist from a nearby hospital reads the x-ray for the physician's office. What modifier is assigned to the services of the physician's office?

a. −26: Professional component

b. −52: Reduced services

c. −Q6: Service furnished by a locum tenens physician

d. −TC: Technical component

30. The surgeon repairs a fistula between the rectum and the anus by placing a graft of OASIS into the wound. How is this service coded?

46280	Surgical treatment of anal fistula (fistulectomy/fistulotomy); transsphincteric, suprasphincteric, extra sphincteric or multiple, including placement of seton, when performed
46288	Closure of anal fistula with rectal advancement flap
46706	Repair of anal fistula with fibrin glue
46707	Repair of anorectal fistula with plug (eg, porcine small intestine submucosa [SIS])

a. 46707

b. 46280

c. 46288

d. 46707, 46706

31. When coding repairs of multiple lacerations in CPT, what action should the coder take?

    a. Code only the most complex repair

    b. Code only the least complex repair

    c. Code all the laceration repairs, listing the most complex repair first

    d. Code all the repairs of the same site using the code for the most complex repair

32. After completing a quality audit on this patient encounter summary, what action should the coding supervisor take?

    Patient Encounter Summary
    Dr. Dunn, Primary Care
    Patient #784309

Date of Service	CPT Code	Description	Diagnosis	Charge
5/1/20XX	73610	X-ray, ankle, complete	719.47	$76.00
5/1/20XX	27816	Closed treatment trimalleolar ankle fracture without manipulation	824.6	$249.00
5/1/20XX	Q4038	Cast supplies, short leg adult fiberglass	824.6	$43.00
5/1/20XX	29405	Cast application, short leg	824.6	$65.00

    a. Clarify the fracture treatment with the physician.

    b. Instruct the physician about proper coding of cast applications.

    c. Instruct the physician to add an office visit.

    d. Query the physician about the correct diagnosis.

33. What is the best reference tool to use when determining how CPT codes should be assigned?

    a. Local coverage determination from Medicare

    b. American Medical Association's CPT Assistant newsletter

    c. American Hospital Association's Coding Clinic

    d. CMS Web site

34. The patient has an imaging study done of the brain where tomographic pictures are taken and a computer is used to reassemble the images. Images are taken before and after dye is injected. The images are interpreted by the physician. How is this service coded?

70450	Computed tomography, head or brain; without contrast material
70460	with contrast material(s)
70470	without contrast material, followed by contrast material(s) and further sections
78607	Brain imaging, tomographic (SPECT)

    a. 70450

    b. 70450, 70460

    c. 70470

    d. 78607

35. The physician provides 115 minutes of critical care to the patient and documents the time in the record. How is this service coded?

99291	Critical care, evaluation and management of the critically ill or critically injured patient; first 30 to 74 minutes
99292	each additional 30 minutes (List separately in addition to code for primary service.)

   a. 99291

   b. 99291, 99292

   c. 99291, 99292, 99292

   d. 99291, 99292, 99292, 99292

36. The physician performs a procedure that cannot be described with a regular code in CPT so an unlisted code is assigned. The physician wants a –22 modifier applied to the code. What is the best action for the coder to take?

   a. Apply the –22 modifier to the unlisted code as requested by the physician

   b. Explain to the physician that modifiers cannot be used on unlisted codes

   c. Submit a different CPT code that describes a lesser procedure and add a –22 modifier

   d. Submit a different CPT code that describes a more extensive procedure and add a –52 modifier

Domain 4: Reimbursement

37. The physician is a participating provider (PAR) whose usual fee for a service provided is $150. The Medicare PAR fee is $130. The patient has met the annual Part B deductible. How much reimbursement does the physician expect to receive from the federal government?

   a. $150

   b. $130

   c. $120

   d. $104

38. The physician is a nonparticipating provider (non-PAR) who accepts assignment. The usual fee for a service rendered is $110. The Medicare PAR fee is $100. Assuming that the Part B deductible has been met, how much reimbursement does the physician expect to receive from the federal government?

   a. $100

   b. $95

   c. $80

   d. $76

39. In the preceding situation, how much does the physician receive from the patient?

    a. $0

    b. $14

    c. $19

    d. $20

40. What is the approved amount for CPT code 99217, Observation Care Discharge with the following values?

wRVU = 1.00
peRVU = 0.5
mRVU = 0.02
wGPCI = 1.0
peGPCI = 1.5
mGPCI = 1.0
CF = $36.0666

    a. $54.82

    b. $63.84

    c. $129.50

    d. $181.05

41. The physician is a non-PAR who does not accept assignment. His usual fee for a service is $200. Medicare's PAR fee is $175. How much can the physician expect to receive from the government, assuming the patient has met the Part B deductible?

    a. $200

    b. $175

    c. $166.25

    d. $0

42. The physician is a non-PAR who does not accept assignment. His usual fee for a service is $200. Medicare's PAR fee is $175. What is Medicare's limiting charge amount?

    a. $200

    b. $191.18

    c. $175

    d. $166.25

43. Which relative value unit reflects the overhead costs involved in providing a service from a physician to a patient?

    a. Work

    b. Practice expense

    c. Malpractice expense

    d. Geographic adjustment factor

44. Within how many days after a claim is denied does a provider have to request a review of that claim?

    a. 30

    b. 60

    c. 90

    d. 120

45. The patient had a total abdominal hysterectomy with bilateral salpingo-oophorectomy. The coder selected the following codes:

58150	Total abdominal hysterectomy, with/without removal of tubes and ovaries
58700	Salpingectomy, complete or partial, unilateral/bilateral (separate procedure)

    What error has the coder made by using these codes?

    a. Maximizing

    b. Upcoding

    c. Unbundling

    d. Optimizing

Domain 5: Data Quality and Analysis

46. After comparing this patient encounter summary and the progress note, where does the coding manager find that education is needed?

    Progress Note for 5-1-20XX

    S This 10-year-old fell on the playground, cutting his right hand.

    O There is a superficial palmar laceration measuring 2.0 cm.

    A 2.0 cm palmer laceration, washed with Betadine, anesthetized with 1% lidocaine and closed with one simple stitch of 5-0 nylon. Triple antibiotic ointment applied.

    P Suture removal in 1 week.

    Patient Encounter Summary

Date	CPT Code	Description	Diagnosis	Description
5-1-20XX	13131	Repair, complex, hand, complex, 1.1 cm to 2.5 cm	882.0	Palm laceration
5-1-20XX	99212	Office visit	882.0	Palm laceration

    a. A higher level of office visit should have been coded.

    b. A –59 modifier should have been added to the office visit.

    c. The documentation does not support the codes assigned.

    d. The local anesthetic should have been coded.

47. A new physician submits four encounters from his first day in clinic. They were all completed incorrectly because a procedure was performed with an E/M visit. What is the best action for the coder to take to resolve the situation for the future?

    a. Recode the charges and then submit them

    b. Educate the physician about the appropriate use of the –25 modifier and the surgical package reporting guidelines

    c. Ask the office manager to inform the physician that procedures are not performed in the office setting

    d. Refuse to process charges until the physician receives formal training

48. Which of the following is the best source of information on what should be included on a new encounter form?

    a. Office manager's opinion

    b. Physician's request

    c. Report of codes assigned in the past year

    d. CPT book section for the specialty of the physician

49. A 1-year-old patient presents to the pediatrician for a physical, MMR, and varicella vaccinations. After reviewing the following coding in an audit, what audit findings did the coding manager determine?

    Patient: Jane Doe
    DOB: 2-28-2006

Date of Service	CPT Code	Description	Diagnosis	Description
2-28-2007	99392	Periodic comprehensive preventive medicine; early childhood (age 1 through 4 years)	V20.2	Routine infant or child health check
2-28-2007	90707	Measles, mumps and rubella virus vaccine (MMR), live, for subcutaneous use	V20.2	Routine infant or child health check
2-28-2007	90716	Varicella virus vaccine, live, for subcutaneous use	V20.2	Routine infant or child health check

    a. The CPT code(s) are incorrect.

    b. The ICD-9-CM code(s) are incorrect.

    c. CPT code(s) are missing.

    d. The case is coded correctly.

50. Which report contains a summary of all billing data entered for a physician's practice for one day, listing all vital pieces of data to be included on the billing form?

    a. Claim history

    b. Diagnosis distribution

    c. Charge summary report

    d. Frequency distribution

51. During a recent audit, the coding manager compared an inventory report and the coding report for the same period. The findings included that the practice had purchased 25 wrist splints and had coded 15 wrist splints during the month. The supply is now gone. What action should the coding manager take?

    a. Talk to the physician(s) about the use of supplies

    b. Ask the Office Manager to evaluate why the counts don't match

    c. Reeducate the staff and physician(s) about supply coding

    d. Suggest that splints no longer be provided by the office

Domain 6: Information and Communication Technologies

52. What is the computer-based transmission of data in a standardized format between providers and third-party payers called?

    a. Electronic claims processing

    b. Common language interchange

    c. Computer language interchange

    d. Electronic data interchange

53. A physician would like to post policy statements and employee manuals electronically in order to enable his employees to have updated reference tools with search capabilities. He wants to make certain that the information is available only to his employees. What electronic tool would he use?

    a. Internet

    b. Extranet

    c. Intranet

    d. Virtual private network

54. What term is used to describe the ability of different information systems to communicate with each other?

    a. Encryption

    b. Interoperability

    c. Functional strategy

    d. Integrated delivery

Domain 7: Compliance and Regulatory Issues

55. The specific legislation that provides for criminal penalties for healthcare professionals who "knowingly and willfully" attempt to defraud any of the healthcare benefit programs and further stipulates that physicians or other providers are accountable for information they "know or should know" is the:

    a. Federal False Claims Act

    b. Health Insurance Portability and Accountability Act

    c. Operation Restore Trust

    d. Balanced Budget Act of 1997

56. The governmental agency that develops an annual "work plan" that delineates the specific target areas that will be monitored in a given year is the:

    a. Federal Bureau of Investigation

    b. Defense Criminal Investigative Service

    c. Office of the Inspector General

    d. U.S. Attorneys' Offices

57. Which of the following is an example of fraud?

    a. Inadvertent filing of duplicate claims

    b. Failure to document medical records adequately

    c. Paying or receiving remuneration or kickbacks for referrals

    d. Failure to comply with a particular agreement

58. A program unveiled by the Office of the Inspector General that expanded and simplified methods for healthcare providers to voluntarily report fraudulent conduct affecting Medicare, Medicaid, and other federal healthcare programs is the:

    a. Provider Self-Disclosure Protocol

    b. Federal False Claims Act

    c. Operation Restore Trust

    d. Health Insurance Portability and Accountability Act

59. The term that refers to the degree to which codes accurately reflect the patient's diagnoses and procedures during a coding audit is:

    a. Reliability

    b. Completeness

    c. Timeliness

    d. Validity

60. Legislation that prohibits physicians from referring Medicare patients to a clinical laboratory in which he or she or an immediate family member has a financial interest is referred to as the:

    a. Kennedy-Kasselbaum Act

    b. Stark Law

    c. Tax Equity and Fiscal Responsibility Act

    d. Provider Self-Disclosure Protocol

Practice Exam 3 Medical Cases

CASE STUDY 1

Please code for the services of the physician.

Practice Exam 3

CASE 1

HISTORY: Follow-up decompression laminectomy and extension of fusion lumbar spine L2 to sacrum performed 1 year ago. Patient generally doing pretty well with back, has achy back discomfort. Main problem is bilateral lateral hip pain. She has a previous diagnosis of trochanteric bursitis. She also describes triggering of her right middle finger with catching of the finger in flexion. The patient had a right knee replacement several years previously.

PHYSICAL EXAMINATION:

VITAL SIGNS: Blood Pressure 137/77. Pulse 79. Temperature is 98.1.

HEENT: Normal

CHEST: Clear

HEART: Normal sinus rhythm, no murmur

SPINE EXAMINATION: Reveals well-healed incision lumbar spine with minimal tenderness, no paravertebral spasm. Range of motion 80% of normal.

HIP EXAMINATION: Reveals full range of motion of hips bilaterally. There is exquisite tenderness over abductor insertion on greater trochanter.

HAND EXAMINATION: Reveals triggering of the right middle finger.

RADIOGRAPHS: Previous x-rays of lumbar spine reviewed showing excellent instrumented fusion L2 to sacrum with fusion consolidation. Extensive narrowing of the spine at the T3-T4 region.

IMPRESSION:
1. Stenosis in thoracic spinal area
2. Bilateral trochanteric bursitis
3. Right middle trigger finger

PLAN:

1. Trochanteric bursa is injected bilateral today under sterile conditions using 5 cc of Kenalog

2. Right middle finger injected today with improvement with 0.5 cc of Kenalog

3. Flexeril 10 mg p.o. t.i.d. p.r.n. Renew hydrocodone 5/500 1 p.o. q.6 h p.r.n. pain

4. Consider surgery on stenosed thoracic region of the spine

5. Return in 6 months' time for reevaluation

HISTORY: Expanded problem-focused

EXAMINATION: Detailed

MEDICAL DECISION-MAKING: Moderate

Answer Sheet

Directions: Be sure to enter all medical record codes in the manner provided in the sample below, paying special attention to the decimal placement for each code. The codes must be typed on the answer sheet in the boxes provided on the computer screen using the keyboard. A decimal point (.) has been provided as a guide for entering each ICD-9-CM code. **You will lose credit if the digits of the codes are correct, but the decimal point has been incorrectly placed.**

CASE 1 DIAGNOSES   **ICD-9-CM**

DX1				.		
DX2				.		
DX3				.		
DX4				.		

CASE 1 PROCEDURES   **CPT/HCPCS**

PR1					
PR2					
PR3					
PR4					
PR5					
PR6					

CASE STUDY 2

Please code for the services of the physician.

Practice Exam 3

CASE 2

DATE OF SERVICE: 12/29/20XX

CHIEF COMPLAINT: Acute left-sided weakness

HISTORY OF PRESENT ILLNESS: The patient is a 47-year-old woman who was on the phone talking to a friend when she had acute weakness to her left arm and left leg. She states her leg and arm felt like an extremity feels when you sleep on it. There was decreased strength, but she states the symptoms and also the sensation is slightly decreased. Her husband noted some slight slurring of her speech. The patient denies any visual changes, loss of vision, double vision. She has not had any headache. She gives no history of any chest pain or palpitations. She presents here stating that her symptoms have somewhat improved.

PAST MEDICAL AND SURGICAL HISTORY:

1. Appendectomy
2. Mitral valve prolapse

CURRENT MEDICATIONS: Ranitidine

SOCIAL HISTORY: She does not smoke. She is a missionary. She has no primary care provider.

FAMILY HISTORY: Negative for early stroke or coronary artery disease.

REVIEW OF SYSTEMS: See HPI, otherwise negative.

PHYSICAL EXAMINATION:

VITAL SIGNS: Temperature 98.1, blood pressure 120/69, pulse 76 and regular, respirations 17, saturation 99% on room air

GENERAL: Awake, alert, nontoxic-appearing female

HEENT: Head is atraumatic, normocephalic. Pupils are equal and round. Extraocular muscles are intact. Cranial nerves II-XII are intact. The palate raises symmetrically.

NECK: Supple, no JVD, no bruits

CHEST: Clear and equal breath sounds bilaterally without any wheezes, rales, or rhonchi

CARDIOVASCULAR: S1 and S2 normal. Regular rate and rhythm. Occasional ectopic beat is noted. I do not appreciate any murmur.

ABDOMEN: Soft

EXTREMITIES: Warm and dry, well perfused

NEUROLOGICAL: She is awake, alert, oriented ×3. Her strength is 5/5 and symmetric. Finger-to-nose normal. Heel-to-shin normal.

EMERGENCY DEPARTMENT COURSE: The patient underwent extensive diagnostics. A continuous three-lead monitor demonstrated a sinus rhythm with occasional PVC. Twelve-lead electrocardiogram revealed a sinus rhythm, occasional PVC, no ST-segment elevation or depression. CT scan of her head was found to be unremarkable. Her white blood cell count was 4.7, normal hemoglobin and hematocrit, normal differential. Comprehensive metabolic and CK were all normal as well. The patient was given aspirin orally here in the department. Given that she is 47 years of age, has mitral valve prolapse, and has rather classic symptoms of a TIA and thought to be at high risk, the patient will be placed in the hospital for further inpatient workup for acute transient ischemic attack, which appears to be improved.

DIAGNOSES:
1. Acute transient ischemic attack
2. Mitral valve prolapse by history

INSTRUCTIONS: The patient's case was discussed with cardiology. The patient will be admitted to a telemetry bed for further care and treatment.

HISTORY: Comprehensive

EXAMINATION: Comprehensive

MEDICAL DECISION-MAKING: High

Answer Sheet

Directions: Be sure to enter all medical record codes in the manner provided in the sample below, paying special attention to the decimal placement for each code. The codes must be typed on the answer sheet in the boxes provided on the computer screen using the keyboard. A decimal point (.) has been provided as a guide for entering each ICD-9-CM code. **You will lose credit if the digits of the codes are correct, but the decimal point has been incorrectly placed.**

CASE 2 DIAGNOSES   **ICD-9-CM**

DX1				.		
DX2				.		
DX3				.		
DX4				.		

CASE 2 PROCEDURES   **CPT/HCPCS**

PR1					
PR2					
PR3					
PR4					
PR5					
PR6					

CASE STUDY 3

Please code for the services of the physician.

Practice Exam 3 CASE 3

CONSULT REQUESTED BY: Dr. A

HISTORY: The patient is a 33-year-old woman who has had known gallstones and post-prandial right upper quadrant and epigastric pain for the last 3 years. She describes the pain as intense gas pains. The pain radiates occasionally to her back. She notes that her pain is worse with fatty food. She has tried herbal remedies without success. She has no history of jaundice or pancreatitis. She has had no emergency department visits or hospitalizations for the pain. The pain is worsening and the patient is sent here for evaluation and definitive diagnosis.

PAST MEDICAL HISTORY:

1. Iron deficiency anemia

PAST SURGICAL HISTORY: None

ALLERGIES: Penicillin

MEDICATIONS:

1. Multivitamins
2. Iron 65 mg, two daily

FAMILY HISTORY: The patient's paternal grandmother had breast cancer. Her paternal grandfather had colon cancer. Her maternal grandfather had lung cancer. Diabetes and hypertension also run in her family.

REVIEW OF SYSTEMS: A 14-point review of systems was completed by the patient today in the office. The patient reports weight gain as well as back pain. She denies any chest pain, shortness of breath, or dysuria. The remaining review of systems is negative.

SOCIAL HISTORY: The patient is married. She works as a managed care coordinator. She does not smoke. She drinks alcohol occasionally.

PHYSICAL EXAMINATION:

VITAL SIGNS: Weight 229.4 pounds. Blood pressure 129/72. Heart rate is 86. Temperature 97.5.

GENERAL: The patient is a pleasant female in no acute distress. Alert and oriented times three.

HEENT: There is no jaundice, thyroid masses, or cervical lymphadenopathy.

RESPIRATORY: Lung sounds are clear bilaterally

HEART: Regular rate and rhythm

ABDOMEN: Soft and nontender. There are no scars or hernias.

MUSCULOSKELETAL: Gait, strength, and muscle tone within normal limits

NEUROLOGIC: Cranial nerves II-XII are grossly intact

DATA: Abdominal ultrasound report shows the gallbladder was markedly contracted with multiple stones. The common bile duct measured 6 mm in diameter.

LABORATORY: Laboratory dated 11/22/20XX, bilirubin 0.2, AST 20, ALT 28, alkaline phosphatase 29, amylase 62, lipase 21

ASSESSMENT/PLAN:

The patient is a 33-year-old otherwise healthy woman with classic symptoms of biliary colic. We had an extensive discussion with the patient in regard to the technical aspects of the laparoscopic cholecystectomy. We discussed the potential complications of the surgery that include but are not limited to: need to convert to open surgery, retained stone, bile duct injury, bleeding, infection, DVT, and pneumonia. All of her questions were answered to her satisfaction. Because of the frequency of her pain, she is eager to proceed with surgery. We have tentatively scheduled her surgery for December 13th. If she develops any questions or concerns, she should call the office.

HISTORY: Comprehensive

EXAMINATION: Comprehensive

MEDICAL DECISION MAKING: Moderate

Answer Sheet

Directions: Be sure to enter all medical record codes in the manner provided in the sample below, paying special attention to the decimal placement for each code. The codes must be typed on the answer sheet in the boxes provided on the computer screen using the keyboard. A decimal point (.) has been provided as a guide for entering each ICD-9-CM code. **You will lose credit if the digits of the codes are correct, but the decimal point has been incorrectly placed.**

CASE 3 DIAGNOSES   **ICD-9-CM**

				.		
DX1				.		
DX2				.		
DX3				.		
DX4				.		

CASE 3 PROCEDURES   **CPT/HCPCS**

PR1					
PR2					
PR3					
PR4					
PR5					
PR6					

CASE STUDY 4

Please code for the services of the physician.

Practice Exam 3   CASE 4

BRIEF HISTORY: This is a 41-year-old white man who was the helmeted driver of a dirt bike going approximately 45 miles per hour when he hit an embankment and fell and landed on his left side. There was no loss of consciousness. He had a prolonged extrication time of approximately 3 hours per report. He is seen as a trauma consult at approximately 11 p.m. and the accident had happened at 15:15 hours. He is hemodynamically stable, complaining of some back pain, left chest pain, left arm and forearm pain, and left foot pain.

PAST MEDICAL HISTORY:

1. Hypertrophic pyloric stenosis as an infant
2. Multiple feet fractures
3. Vertebral body fractures

MEDICATIONS: None

PAST SURGICAL HISTORY:

1. Left distal radius plating
2. Pylorotomy as an infant

ALLERGIES: No known drug allergies.

FAMILY HISTORY: Unknown because the patient is adopted.

SOCIAL HISTORY: Positive for ETOH approximately one to two drinks per night. Denies any smoking or drugs.

REVIEW OF SYSTEMS: Otherwise negative in general, dermatologic, ear, nose, and throat, cardiovascular, pulmonary, gastrointestinal, genitourinary, psychiatric, neurologic, skin. Positive for history of present illness in the musculoskeletal.

GENERAL: Airway is clear with no intervention needed. C spine is immobilized in a hard collar. Breathing is spontaneous and unlabored.

CIRCULATION: The skin is dry, normal color with no evidence of external hemorrhage.

PULSES: Present at the carotid, radial, and femoral pulses, and dorsalis pedis pulses bilaterally.

DISABILITY: The patient is alert and oriented ×3. GSC of 15. Pupils equal, round, and reactive to light and accommodation measuring 3 mm in diameter.

HEENT: There is not any evidence for any external trauma. Pupils are 3 mm and reactive bilaterally. Gaze is normal. Extraocular movements are intact. Tympanic membranes are clear bilaterally. There is no abnormality of mouth, teeth, or pharynx. Occlusion is normal. No facial bony deformities or crepitus.

NECK: Trachea is midline. No jugular venous distention.

CHEST: There are some mild abrasions of the left lateral chest wall. He has good movement and chest wall is symmetric bilaterally. Breath sounds are clear to auscultation bilaterally.

HEART: Regular rate and rhythm without murmurs, rubs, or gallops. There is no crepitus. There is some mild tenderness to palpation on the left lateral chest wall.

ABDOMEN: There are some abrasions in the left lower quadrant of the abdomen; otherwise the abdomen is soft, nontender, nondistended with good bowel sounds.

PELVIS: Stable and nontender

GENITOURINARY: There is no blood in the meatus.

RECTAL: Examination is deferred.

SPINE: Cervical spine is nontender to palpation with no obvious step-offs or deformities and full active range of motion. Thoracic spine is tender at the T8 vertebral body area with no obvious step-offs or deformities. Lumbar spine is nontender to palpation.

EXTREMITIES: There is mild tenderness to palpation at the left proximal forearm and left foot approximately at the 4th metatarsal with some mild abrasions over the dorsal aspect of the left forearm. Pulses are present and 3+ of the radial, carotids, femoral, popliteal, posterior tibial and dorsalis pedis pulses bilaterally.

NEUROLOGIC: 5/5 strength in range of motion all four extremities. Sensation is grossly intact.

AP chest reveals central vascular congestion. No pneumothorax or wide mediastinum. AP pelvis revealed no acute fracture or dislocation. Left forearm films revealed a proximal left ulnar fracture that is minimally displaced and evidence of a previously repaired left radius fracture. CT of the head revealed no acute fracture, dislocation, or intracranial bleed. CT of the cervical spine was negative. CT of the chest reveals right first rib fracture. Multiple left-sided rib fractures and a small hemothorax. CT of the abdomen and pelvis revealed no acute intra-abdominal pathology. Thoracic and lumbar spine reconstruction revealed the T7-8 compression fractures that were old. These were reviewed with Dr. X.

Trauma examination performed in the emergency department was negative in the right upper quadrant and subxiphoid, retropubic area, however, the overall examination was indeterminate because of a poorly visualized perisplenic view.

LABORATORY EXAMINATIONS: Obtained and revealed a hemoglobin of 16.1, sodium 144, potassium 3.6, chloride 101, BUN not an applicable base deficit of -1, pH 7.35, PO_2-39, PCO_2-47, lactate 2.3, glucose 109.

ASSESSMENT: A 41-year-old man status post dirt bike accident with multiple left-sided rib fractures, hemothorax, left ulnar fracture that is closed, and chest wall abrasions. His C spine was cleared clinically in the emergency department.

PLAN: He was admitted for pain control and observation. Will have a repeat chest x-ray and complete blood count in the morning. Abrasions are cleaned, antibiotic ointment applied, and dressed with bandages. Given a PCA and Toradol for pain. Orthopedics department was consulted and the patient will need a simple splint for his left ulnar fracture. Pulmonary consult was requested.

HISTORY: Comprehensive

EXAMINATION: Comprehensive

MEDICAL DECISION-MAKING: High

Answer Sheet

Directions: Be sure to enter all medical record codes in the manner provided in the sample below, paying special attention to the decimal placement for each code. The codes must be typed on the answer sheet in the boxes provided on the computer screen using the keyboard. A decimal point (.) has been provided as a guide for entering each ICD-9-CM code. **You will lose credit if the digits of the codes are correct, but the decimal point has been incorrectly placed.**

CASE 4 DIAGNOSES   **ICD-9-CM**

DX1				.		
DX2				.		
DX3				.		
DX4				.		

CASE 4 PROCEDURES   **CPT/HCPCS**

PR1					
PR2					
PR3					
PR4					
PR5					
PR6					

CASE STUDY 5

Please code for the services of the physician.

Practice Exam 3   CASE 5

REASON FOR VISIT: Patient comes in today for monitoring of his chronic obstructive pulmonary disease, but he is apparently having a flare up that he thinks just started within the last day or so. There has been no fever or chills. He has had cough, but the sputum has been fairly clear. There is no chest pain, but it does feel tight. He has been more dyspneic, particularly with attempts to come to the office today. He's not had any trouble with edema. Patient has long standing CLL.

MEDICATIONS:

1. Oxygen, 3 L/minute via nasal cannula continuously
2. Advair, 250/50, one inhalation q 12 h
3. Combivent, 2 puffs four times daily and as needed
4. Zyrtec, 10 mg daily, as needed
5. Prednisone, 5 mg daily
6. Norvasc, 10 mg daily
7. Tylenol No. 3 as needed

PHYSICAL EXAMINATION:

GENERAL: Pleasant, slightly cushingoid, elderly, white man in no distress, but he is definitely more tachypneic and labored with his speech than usual. WEIGHT: 128. BLOOD PRESSURE: 170/80. PULSE: 88 and regular. RESPIRATIONS: 16 to 18.

NOSE: Nasal mucosa and turbinates clear

MOUTH: Clear

PHARYNX: Clear

NECK: Supple. No cervical or supraclavicular adenopathy.

LUNGS: Bilateral wheezes with poor air movement and prolonged expiratory phase; air movement is not as good as usual.

CARDIAC: Normal S1 and S2; I don't detect an S3

ABDOMEN: No tenderness

EXTREMITIES: No cyanosis, clubbing, or edema

LABORATORY: Oxygen saturation at rest on 3 L of oxygen with a conserver device is 96%. CBC today from laboratory is WNL.

ASSESSMENT/PLAN:

1. COPD/chronic bronchitis, now with moderate exacerbation. Treat with prednisone, 40 mg daily for 3 days then taper by 10 mg every third day; also treat empirically with Levaquin, 750 mg daily for 5 days.

2. Questionable asbestosis based on chest radiographic abnormalities, currently receiving disability compensation

3. Chronic lymphocytic leukemia; will monitor again at next visit

4. Anxiety disorder

HISTORY: Detailed

EXAMINATION: Detailed

MEDICAL DECISION-MAKING: Moderate

Answer Sheet

Directions: Be sure to enter all medical record codes in the manner provided in the sample below, paying special attention to the decimal placement for each code. The codes must be typed on the answer sheet in the boxes provided on the computer screen using the keyboard. A decimal point (.) has been provided as a guide for entering each ICD-9-CM code. **You will lose credit if the digits of the codes are correct, but the decimal point has been incorrectly placed.**

CASE 5 DIAGNOSES   **ICD-9-CM**

DX1				.	
DX2				.	
DX3				.	
DX4				.	

CASE 5 PROCEDURES   **CPT/HCPCS**

PR1					
PR2					
PR3					
PR4					
PR5					
PR6					

CASE STUDY 6

Please code for the services of the physician.

Practice Exam 3 CASE 6

HISTORY OF PRESENT ILLNESS: This is a 4-year-old Hispanic girl who is presenting new to me today and is 6 weeks after a left supracondylar fracture ×3, which occurred on 06/16/20XX status post closed reduction and percutaneous pinning by another physician on 06/17. The patient has Still's syndrome.

X-rays today show a well-healing fracture with pins in place. Long-arm cast was removed today prior to films.

Patient had pain for the first couple days after the injury and after the procedure and then patient denied pain and mom said that she had been complaining of pain after those first couple of days.

PAST MEDICAL HISTORY: She has no past medical history.

MEDICATIONS: No medications

ALLERGIES: No allergies

PHYSICAL EXAMINATION: On examination she has 3 percutaneous pins that are protruding from the dorsal aspect of the elbow. There are no signs of infection, no warmth, redness, or edema. She has normal sensation and motor function of the left hand and 2+ radial pulses.

IMPRESSION: Well-healing supracondylar fracture with percutaneous pins.

PLAN: Pins were removed today in clinic and sterile dressing was applied. We will see this patient back in 4 weeks for follow-up with x-rays at that time. We counseled the mother regarding the limited activity for the patient over the next 4 weeks including no monkey bars, no running, no bicycling, no activity where the patient would be at risk for a fall.

HISTORY: Problem-focused

EXAMINATION: Expanded problem-focused

MEDICAL DECISION-MAKING: Moderate

Answer Sheet

Directions: Be sure to enter all medical record codes in the manner provided in the sample below, paying special attention to the decimal placement for each code. The codes must be typed on the answer sheet in the boxes provided on the computer screen using the keyboard. A decimal point (.) has been provided as a guide for entering each ICD-9-CM code. **You will lose credit if the digits of the codes are correct, but the decimal point has been incorrectly placed.**

CASE 6 DIAGNOSES   **ICD-9-CM**

DX1				.		
DX2				.		
DX3				.		
DX4				.		

CASE 6 PROCEDURES   **CPT/HCPCS**

PR1					
PR2					
PR3					
PR4					
PR5					
PR6					

CASE STUDY 7

Please code for the services of the surgeon.

Practice Exam 3 {CASE 7}

PREOPERATIVE DIAGNOSIS: Right carotid stenosis

POSTOPERATIVE DIAGNOSIS: Right carotid stenosis

PROCEDURE: Right carotid endarterectomy

INDICATION: This patient is a 53-year-old man who was recently hospitalized. During the course of his workup, he was noted to have a right carotid stenosis. This was asymptomatic. Angiography confirmed the finding and it appeared to be approximately 80% stenosis in the right internal carotid artery. The opposite carotid artery is in good condition. The patient was carefully advised about the risks, benefits, and alternatives for asymptomatic carotid stenosis, including the magnitude of reduction of stroke risk in comparison with the actual stroke risk without surgery. The patient understood that this is a purely prophylactic procedure that could cause stroke as a risk and other complications such as tongue paralysis, lower right lip paralysis, numbness in the neck, bleeding, infection, paralysis, and death. He understands the above and requested that surgery be performed.

OPERATIVE COURSE: After general endotracheal anesthesia, the patient was placed in the supine position. The right anterior neck areas were then prepared and draped in the usual fashion. An incision, which was running anterior to the border of the sternocleidomastoid muscles, was made using a #10 blade. Hemostasis was achieved using Bovie, which was used to transverse the platysma. Self-retaining retractors were placed. The plane anterior to the sternocleidomastoid muscle was then developed, using sharp and blunt dissection. Careful hemostasis was employed using bipolar cautery. The carotid sheath was then entered and the carotid and internal jugular veins were dissected out. The Henley retractor was placed. The carotid was dissected distally. There was no obvious common facial vein in the vicinity of the carotid bifurcation which was, as predicted, highly placed. This necessitated careful and deliberate dissection distally, so as to preserve the hypoglossal nerve. This required division of the digastric muscle, using cautery. Great care was taken to identify and preserve the hypoglossal nerve. The need for careful preservation of this was attended to throughout the entire procedure. A small vein that was a tributary to the internal jugular vein was ligated and divided in this area as well.

A Rummel tourniquet was placed around the common carotid artery. 0 silk ties were placed around the internal and external carotid artery, and a 0 silk tie Potts ligature was placed around the first branch of the external carotid artery. There was no typically-placed superior thyroid artery in this patient. It was unclear which branch of the external artery was thus represented as the first proximal branch that was identified. The carotid sinus nerves were infiltrated using 1% lidocaine in the area and the bifurcation was extensively dissected out to allow for placement of these sutures around the vessels. A Hemovac drain was placed lateral to the carotid artery and this was connected to suction. The patient was given 80 units/kg bolus of heparin. The internal, common, and external carotid arteries were test occluded and there was no change in the EEG. The artery was then opened using a #11 blade. This was extended using Potts scissors. The plaque was shelled out in the usual fashion using #4 Penfield. The plaque was amputated proximally in the usual fashion by dividing it with a #11 blade after elevation using a right-angle clamp. The plaque was then removed from the external carotid artery using a standard eversion technique. The plaque was then dissected free at the internal carotid artery distally. An excellent break point was noted and there did not appear to be any need for any intimal tack-up stitches placed.

The arteriotomy bed was then carefully inspected, and all flaky material was removed in standard fashion. The arteriotomy was then closed using running 6-0 Prolene suture. Prior to placement of the final sutures, internal/external carotid arteries were back-bled and heparinized saline was employed to remove any potential bubbles. The external and common were then unclamped, allowing perfusion out this route. The internal was subsequently unclamped, after it had been clamped for a total of 30 minutes. There was no change in the EEG or somatosensory of a potential monitoring during that time or at any other time during the operation. There appeared to be no worthy leakage from the anteriotomy site. The arteries were then inspected at great length with a Doppler to ensure an adequate signal. Thus, satisfied, we proceeded to close. The Hemovac drain was left in place. Great care was taken to ensure excellent hemostasis. In light of this rather atypical amount of ooze present, a partial reversal of the heparin was given by the anesthesiologist. The platysma was then closed using interrupted 2-0 Vicryl sutures. The skin was closed using a running 4-0 Monocryl suture. Steri-Strips and a dressing were applied. The patient was then extubated and taken to the recovery room in stable condition, moving all four extremities well.

Answer Sheet

Directions: Be sure to enter all medical record codes in the manner provided in the sample below, paying special attention to the decimal placement for each code. The codes must be typed on the answer sheet in the boxes provided on the computer screen using the keyboard. A decimal point (.) has been provided as a guide for entering each ICD-9-CM code. **You will lose credit if the digits of the codes are correct, but the decimal point has been incorrectly placed.**

CASE 7 DIAGNOSES   **ICD-9-CM**

					.		
DX1					.		
DX2					.		
DX3					.		
DX4					.		

CASE 7 PROCEDURES   **CPT/HCPCS**

PR1					
PR2					
PR3					
PR4					
PR5					
PR6					

CASE STUDY 8

Please code for the services of the surgeon.

Practice Exam 3

CASE 8

DATE OF OPERATION: 11/08/20XX

PREOPERATIVE DIAGNOSIS: Mucocele, inside right lower lip

POSTOPERATIVE DIAGNOSIS: Mucocele, inside right lower lip

OPERATION: Excision of right lower lip mucocele

ANESTHESIA: General via laryngeal mask airway (LMA)

SPECIMENS: Mucocele from right lower lip

OPERATIVE FINDINGS: Consistent with above

ESTIMATED BLOOD LOSS: Less than 10 mL

COMPLICATIONS: None

INDICATIONS: The patient is a healthy 6-year-old girl who was referred to our clinic from an outside medical clinic for evaluation of a lower lip mucocele. This small lesion has been present for several months and is indicated for removal. Prior to going to the operating room, the details of the procedure along with all risks and all questions were invited and answered with the mother with interpreter present. They elected to have this procedure performed in the operating room under general anesthesia.

PROCEDURE: The patient was properly identified in the preanesthesia holding area and her consent, NPO status and history and physical examination are updated, reviewed, and verified. At this time she was brought to operating theater #10 where she was placed in the supine position. Next, the anesthesia team induced and intubated the patient without complication. The tube was secured and the patient was maintained under general anesthesia throughout the entire procedure. At this time a time-out and patient and procedure verification took place. Next, the patient was prepared, draped, and padded in the usual fashion for a procedure of this type. At this time approximately 2 cc of 0.25% Marcaine with epinephrine 1:200,000 was infiltrated in the right lower lip in the area of the medial nerve. Next, a #15 blade was used to make an elliptical incision around the 3 mm × 3 mm mucocele on the inside of the right lower lip. This was taken just through mucosa. Next, a superficial submucosal dissection was undertaken and the mucocele was removed in its entirety. The surgeon was careful to remain just under the mucosa so that no damage to the medial nerve or its branches would take place. Following this, the wound was irrigated and closed with 5-0 Vicryl in multiple running horizontal mattress sutures. The patient was then awakened, extubated, and taken to the postanesthesia care unit (PACU) in stable condition. There were no complications. All sponge and needle counts were correct ×2.

Pathology Report

CLINICAL INFORMATION:

PROCEDURE: Excision of mucocele lower lip

PREOP DIAGNOSIS: Mucocele lower lip

CLINICAL HISTORY: Not given

GROSS DESCRIPTION:

Received in formalin for routine examination designated MUCOCELE RIGHT LOWER LIP are two fragments of tissue measuring 0.6 cm and 0.2 cm in maximal dimension. The tissue is wrapped and entirely submitted in one cassette.

MICROSCOPIC DESCRIPTION:

Sections contain oral epithelium with underlying glandular tissue that has both serous and acinar cells. The gland has intact architecture, although lumen of the excretory duct is dilated. The stroma immediately under the oral epithelium contains an irregularly shaped cystic space that contains proteinaceous fluid and neutrophils. The adjacent stroma contains reactive capillaries and venules with mild chronic inflammation. No definite mucous is present. Additional step sections were examined.

DIAGNOSIS:

ORAL MUCOSA, LOWER LIP, EXCISION: MUCOUS RETENTION CYST

Answer Sheet

Directions: Be sure to enter all medical record codes in the manner provided in the sample below, paying special attention to the decimal placement for each code. The codes must be typed on the answer sheet in the boxes provided on the computer screen using the keyboard. A decimal point (.) has been provided as a guide for entering each ICD-9-CM code. **You will lose credit if the digits of the codes are correct, but the decimal point has been incorrectly placed.**

CASE 8 DIAGNOSES   **ICD-9-CM**

DX1				.		
DX2				.		
DX3				.		
DX4				.		

CASE 8 PROCEDURES   **CPT/HCPCS**

PR1					
PR2					
PR3					
PR4					
PR5					
PR6					

CASE STUDY 9

Please code for the services of the surgeon.

Practice Exam 3 CASE 9

DATE OF OPERATION: 12/08/20XX

PREOPERATIVE DIAGNOSES:

1. Stage IV metastatic renal cell carcinoma
2. Metastatic disease involving the left femoral neck, left peritrochanteric proximal femur with nondisplaced pathologic fracture of the neck of the femur
3. Metastatic disease involving the left supracondylar femur with impending pathologic fracture

PROCEDURE:

1. Resection of the left femoral head and metastatic neck, renal cell carcinoma
2. Long-stem cemented hemiarthroplasty utilizing the Smith & Nephew Echelon cemented 175-mm #12 stem with a 48-mm 0 neck endo-head
3. Extended curettage and methylmethaculate of the left supracondylar femur
4. Open reduction internal fixation of left distal femur utilizing a Synthes nine-hole 3.5 plate and screws

ANESTHESIA: General

ESTIMATED BLOOD LOSS: For the distal femur was less than 50 cc. For the hip was 150 cc.

INDICATIONS FOR PROCEDURE: This is a 58-year-old man in whom a large renal cell carcinoma was diagnosed earlier this year, has undergone multiple other orthopedic procedures for bone disease, has had radiation therapy for a subtrochanteric lesion in the left femur, developed a new lytic lesion in the femoral neck, has gone on to progression and pain. Additionally, he was noted to have a separate discrete lesion in the distal supracondylar femur on the left. After preoperative embolization performed yesterday, the patient is brought to the operating room for the above-stated surgical procedures.

FINDINGS AT SURGERY: At the time of surgery, the left distal femur underwent an eventful curettage, methylmethaculate and open reduction internal fixation, given very stable fixation, ready for immediate weightbearing. The patient's proximal left femur was noted to have a nondisplaced but complete fracture at the base of the neck, therefore is not deemed a candidate for a spiral blade intermedullary fixation and therefore opted for a head and neck resection followed by a long-stemmed cemented hemiarthroplasty that also gave a very stable and excellent fixation ready for immediate weightbearing.

DESCRIPTION OF PROCEDURE: The patient was identified, brought to the operating room, placed on the operating room table in the supine position where general anesthesia was induced. The patient was oroendotracheally intubated. After he was stabilized, he was carefully and gently placed on the O.S.I. fracture table with a bump beneath the left hip. He received antibiotic prophylaxis and the left hindquarter was prepared and draped in the usual sterile fashion. Under C-arm fluoroscopy, we ranged his hip and noted that the femoral head was not moving in unison with the femoral neck and therefore opted out of antegrade inter-medullary nailing. We therefore proceeded with the distal femur first, which was approached with a direct lateral approach to the femur. The vastus lateralis was elevated. The underlying lytic lesion, which measured approximately 2 cm × 4 cm, was identified, entered with a sharp knife, then a burr, curetted extensively throughout the intermedullary canal back to normal cortical bone. This was irrigated and dried with peroxide and saline. Methylmethaculate was mixed to a doughy state, digitally impacted to fill this defect. A nine-hole 3.5 Synthes plate was then bent and twisted to contour the lateral femur and fixed in the usual standard fashion with 35 screws. This gave excellent rigid fixation. Routine closure was obtained utilizing 0, 2-0 Vicryl followed by skin staples and sterile Tegaderm.

At this time the patient was again prepared and draped in the right lateral decubitus position with care taken to pad bony prominences, neurovascular structures for a posterior approach to his left hip. Through a standard posterolateral approach to his hip, the proximal femur was identified, hip arthrotomy performed, and findings as noted above osteotomizing the proximal femur just above the lesser trochanter. Femoral head and neck were excised, were extensively involved with malignancy. These were passed off as specimen. The proximal femur was curetted back to stable bone. Then it was reamed and broached to accept a 175-mm, #12 stem. Length was verified as satisfactory under C-arm fluoroscopy. The canal was prepared, dried, distal cement restrictor placed and the #12 stem was cemented into standard anteversion utilizing excellent cement technique. After it had dried, a 48-mm 0 neck was impacted onto the prosthesis having been previously measured. This was reduced and noted to give excellent stable reduction. The wound was then copiously irrigated with antibiotic-containing saline solution and closed with 0 Vicryl interrupted, short external rotators reattached to the gluteus medius tendon, fascia closed with 0 Vicryl interrupted, 2-0 Vicryl inverted and skin staples. A medium Hemovac drain was used in the hip wound.

The patient was then returned to the supine position, awakened and extubated in the operating room, moved to the recovery room in stable condition.

POSTOPERATIVE PLAN: For routine posterior hip precautions, weightbearing as tolerated.

Answer Sheet

Directions: Be sure to enter all medical record codes in the manner provided in the sample below, paying special attention to the decimal placement for each code. The codes must be typed on the answer sheet in the boxes provided on the computer screen using the keyboard. A decimal point (.) has been provided as a guide for entering each ICD-9-CM code. **You will lose credit if the digits of the codes are correct, but the decimal point has been incorrectly placed.**

CASE 9 DIAGNOSES   **ICD-9-CM**

DX1				.		
DX2				.		
DX3				.		
DX4				.		

CASE 9 PROCEDURES   **CPT/HCPCS**

PR1					
PR2					
PR3					
PR4					
PR5					
PR6					

CASE STUDY 10

Please code for the services of the surgeon.

Practice Exam 3   CASE 10

DATE OF OPERATION: 11/01/20XX

PREOPERATIVE DIAGNOSIS: Left orbital pseudotumor

POSTOPERATIVE DIAGNOSIS: Left orbital pseudotumor

OPERATION: Anterior orbitotomy with a biopsy of lacrimal gland, left orbit

ANESTHESIA: General

SURGICAL INDICATIONS: The patient is a 10-year-old boy with a 2-year history of chronic inflammation of the left orbit including swelling of the medial and lateral recti muscles and the ipsilateral lacrimal gland and Tenon's capsule. Previous diagnostic studies included a normal CBC, C-reactive protein (less than 0.1), and C-ANCA and P-ANCA, which were negative suggesting there was no underlying vasculitis. Because of continued chronic inflammation for which he will probably need oral steroids, pretreatment biopsy of involved tissue was recommended. Brief review of the CT scan revealed that there was considerable enlargement of the lacrimal gland in the left orbit, therefore biopsy of this tissue was recommended.

SURGICAL PROCEDURE: The child was brought to the operating room after adequate preoperative medications. He was induced with face mask anesthesia at which time an intravenous line was inserted, cardiac monitor, blood pressure cuff, EKG leads, and pulse oximeter were attached. The child was then intubated and maintained with an appropriate combination and mixture of anesthetic gases and oxygen compatible with general surgery. His face was prepared and draped in the usual sterile fashion.

Inspection of the left eyelid revealed that there was no crease. There was proptosis of the ipsilateral globe with fullness of the left upper eyelid. There seemed to be a previous scar in the left upper eyelid. Therefore the decision was made to position the anterior orbitotomy on the previous left upper eyelid scar. Therefore approximately a 2-cm area was demarcated with a marking pen in the superotemporal aspect of the upper eyelid above the area where the eyelid crease would normally be. The subcutaneous tissue was infiltrated with 1% Xylocaine with epinephrine. A #67 Beaver blade was used to incise the eyelid skin and superficial orbicularis. Prior to doing this, the eyelid was put on stretch by putting a 6-0 silk through the lash line and pulling the upper eyelid taut. Then the eyelid skin was tented up with small muscle hooks. The orbicularis muscle was incised centrally and then the incision in the orbicularis was extended to the medial and lateral margins of the skin incision. Hemostasis was obtained with bipolar cautery. The sharp dissection was continued posteriorly to the level of the orbital septum. The area of the orbital septum just at its junction with the lateral orbital rim was exposed using Ragnell retractors. The orbital septum was then incised and retracted. One could immediately see the orbital portion of the lacrimal gland prolapsed through the wound. The pseudocapsule of the lacrimal gland was separated on the posterior aspect of the gland. A small amount of tissue was tented up on a forceps and excised using the #67 Beaver blade. The tissue was immediately sent to the histopathology laboratory as a fresh specimen for appropriate histopathology and immunohistochemistry as indicated. Hemostasis was obtained with digital pressure and topical application of Avitene.

Once hemostasis was obtained, the wound was closed in a two-layered approach. First a deep subcutaneous and orbicularis muscle was closed with 5-0 Vicryl and then the skin was closed with several interrupted 6-0 plain. Topical ointment was placed on the wound. The child was then weaned from general anesthesia, extubated, and brought to the recovery room in good health without complications.

Pathology Report

CLINICAL INFORMATION

PROCEDURE: Biopsy left orbital lesion

PREOPERATIVE DIAGNOSIS: Left orbital lesion

CLINICAL HISTORY: 10-year-old boy with chronic orbital inflammation (eye muscles, lacrimal gland) for 2 years

GROSS DESCRIPTION:

Received fresh designated LEFT LACRIMAL GLAND is a single, unoriented, irregular tan-pink portion of soft tissue measuring 0.8 × 0.6 × 0.1 cm, which is submitted entirely, intact, in one cassette.

MICROSCOPIC DESCRIPTION:

H&E-stained sections reveal a portion of lacrimal tissue, with well-organized lobules of glands separated by fibromuscular tissue bands. Occasional ducts are seen within the fibromuscular tissue. Scattered collections of lymphocytes, plasma cells, and eosinophils are present between the exocrine glands and in foci within the intervening fibrous bands. There is no evidence of a neoplastic process.

DIAGNOSIS:

LEFT LACRIMAL GLAND, BIOPSY; LACRIMAL GLAND TISSUE WITH AT MOST MILDLY INCREASED INTERSTITIAL LYMPHOCYTES AND PLASMA CELLS (SEE COMMENT)

COMMENT:

Normal lacrimal gland tissue contains scattered interstitial lymphocytes and plasma cells. The number of lymphocytes and plasma cells present in this biopsy are, at most, mildly increased. An infiltrative or neoplastic cell population is not identified.

Answer Sheet

Directions: Be sure to enter all medical record codes in the manner provided in the sample below, paying special attention to the decimal placement for each code. The codes must be typed on the answer sheet in the boxes provided on the computer screen using the keyboard. A decimal point (.) has been provided as a guide for entering each ICD-9-CM code. **You will lose credit if the digits of the codes are correct, but the decimal point has been incorrectly placed.**

CASE 10 DIAGNOSES   ICD-9-CM

DX1				.		
DX2				.		
DX3				.		
DX4				.		

CASE 10 PROCEDURES   CPT/HCPCS

PR1					
PR2					
PR3					
PR4					
PR5					
PR6					

CASE STUDY 11

Please code for the services of the surgeon.

Practice Exam 3   CASE 11

DATE OF OPERATION: 12/15/20XX

PREOPERATIVE DIAGNOSIS: Right middle ear cholesteatoma

POSTOPERATIVE DIAGNOSIS: Right middle ear cholesteatoma

OPERATION: Right mastoidectomy, tympanoplasty

FINDINGS: Cholesteatoma, right anterior middle ear epitympanum, intact ossicular chain

INDICATIONS: The patient is an 18-year-old woman with previous ear surgery elsewhere and then a right tympanoplasty here in 2001 for anterior-superior middle ear cholesteatoma. She was seen recently with enlarging right anterior-superior whitish mass within the tympanic membrane.

OPERATIVE PROCEDURE: After endotracheal intubation and administration of general anesthesia, the right ear was prepared and draped in the usual fashion. The ear was inspected with a microscope. The patient was known to have a whitish mass within an intact tympanic membrane in the anterior-superior quadrant of the middle ear. A canal incision was made 4 mm behind the posterior bony annulus with a 7200 blade from 6 o'clock to 12 o'clock. A postauricular incision was made with a 15-blade knife, and the periosteum was divided under the linea temporalis and behind the ear canal. At this point, the patient was found to have no accessible temporalis fascia. The temporalis muscle was then retracted superiorly with a Senn rake, and a 1.5 cm × 1.5 cm periosteal graft was harvested from underneath the temporalis fascia. This was cleaned and placed on the Mayo stand for drying. The ear canal was brought forward with a Freer elevator down to the previously made incision.

At this point, the patient was known to have a cholesteatoma that was within the posterior-superior ear canal in an area of scalloped-out bone. This cholesteatoma pearl was removed with a duckbill and then stapes curet. This was not contiguous with any other process. The tympanomeatal flap was elevated down to bony annulus, and then the middle ear was entered under the membranous annulus with a Rosen needle and annulus elevator. It was reflected forward to the malleus handle. At this point, the patient was known to have cholesteatoma extending along the medial surface of the malleus handle and body of malleus involving the anterior portion of tensor tympani tendon and filling the entire anterior middle ear and anterior epitympanum. The tympanic membrane was dissected off the malleus handle in its entirety with a 5910 Beaver blade and then reflected up to the anterior ear canal. The cholesteatoma mass was removed from the anterior hypotympanum, anterior-superior middle ear, and anterior epitypanum with a combination of duckbills and cupped forceps. It was difficult to visualize the tensor tympani tendon. The tensor tympani tendon was therefore cut at its attachment to the neck of the malleus with a 5910 blade and, with gentle lateral retraction on the malleus, the cholesteatoma could be followed up and dissected off the anterior surface of the body of the malleus. At this point, no other cholesteatoma was noted in the middle ear or epitympanum.

A mastoidectomy was carried out by removing the lateral cortex with a 3-mm burr to expose the posterior epitympanum. Dissection was carried further up to the short process of the malleus with a stapes curet. The mucosa in the posterior epitympanum was clean. No other cholesteatoma was noted under the incus. Irrigation at that point flowed freely over the facial ridge into the middle ear.

Next, the middle ear was inspected again. A small amount of granulation tissue was dissected from around the long process of the incus and the incudostapedial joint, which was intact. No cholesteatoma was noted in that area. At this point, inspection of the middle ear and epitympanum yielded no evidence of recurrent cholesteatoma. A portion of the anterior tympanic membrane from the malleus handle up to the annulus was resected, where that had been contiguous with the main portion of the inflamed cholesteatoma mass. This resulted in about a 35% anterior marginal perforation. The anterior annulus was raised at the level of the perforation with a round 90-degree canal knife, and a Rosen needle was then used to make an adjacent tunnel under anterior ear canal skin. The previously harvested periosteal graft was placed under the malleus handle so that the anterior edge was positioned just at the mouth of the eustachian tube. A microcup forceps was placed into the previously made tunnel and the anterior edge of the graft was pulled up anterior and underneath the anterior membranous annulus in order to hold the graft in place on the anterior canal wall. The posterior aspect of the graft and the tympanomeatal flap were reflected forward, and several pieces of Gelfoam were placed in the middle ear and pushed forward into the middle ear, instilled with Gelfoam, and the graft was elevated to meet the surrounding tympanic membrane. The posterior aspect of the graft was placed on the posterior ear canal along the remainder of the tympanomeatal flap, and Gelfoam was placed starting anteriorly to reconstitute the anterior sulcus and then over the entire tympanic membrane and graft.

The postauricular incision was closed in three layers with periosteum, auricular muscle, and dermis with 3-0 and 4-0 chromic. Steri-Strips were applied, and Gelfoam was then used to pack the remainder of the external ear canal. Estimated blood loss was approximately 100 cc. The final status of the middle ear is intact mobile ossicular chain, medial periosteal graft to anterior marginal 35% perforation.

PLAN: I explained to the patient's parents that if we get a significant recurrence along the ossicles, then the plan in the future will probably be to divide the incudostapedial joint and remove the head of the malleus and incus for better access to the epitympanum.

Answer Sheet

Directions: Be sure to enter all medical record codes in the manner provided in the sample below, paying special attention to the decimal placement for each code. The codes must be typed on the answer sheet in the boxes provided on the computer screen using the keyboard. A decimal point (.) has been provided as a guide for entering each ICD-9-CM code. **You will lose credit if the digits of the codes are correct, but the decimal point has been incorrectly placed.**

CASE 11 DIAGNOSES   **ICD-9-CM**

					.		
DX1					.		
DX2					.		
DX3					.		
DX4					.		

CASE 11 PROCEDURES   **CPT/HCPCS**

PR1					
PR2					
PR3					
PR4					
PR5					
PR6					

CASE STUDY 12

Please code for the services of the surgeon.

Practice Exam 3   CASE 12

SERVICE: Abdominal transplant

PREOPERATIVE DIAGNOSES: Persistent rejection and failed renal allograft with allograft nephropathy resulting in end-stage renal disease

POSTOPERATIVE DIAGNOSES: Persistent rejection and failed renal allograft with allograft nephropathy resulting in end-stage renal disease

OPERATIONS AND PROCEDURES: Transplant nephrectomy

ANESTHESIA: General endotracheal

INDICATIONS FOR THE OPERATION: The patient is a 25-year-old woman who underwent a kidney transplant that subsequently failed due to persistent rejection. She has met end-stage criteria and is now being dialyzed, however, continues to suffer persistent rejection despite triple immunosuppression. For this reason, she presents to the OR for elective nephrectomy to take care of the above issues and also get her off of immunosuppression.

PROCEDURE: The patient was identified and brought to the operating room and placed in the supine position and administered general endotracheal anesthetic. Her abdomen was shaved, prepared and draped in a sterile fashion. She was explored through her previous right hockey stick incision. This was carried through the layers of the abdominal wall with care to avoid entrance into the peritoneal cavity. The kidney transplant was identified. The capsule was separated freeing the kidney circumferentially down to its vascular pedicle. Large vascular clamps were placed both from a superior and inferior position and crossclamped. The femoral artery pulse was checked and found to be 2+. The kidney was then amputated off its vascular pedicle above the clamps and vessels were secured with two rows of running 3-0 Prolene. Crossclamps were removed and hemostasis was noted with no significant blood loss. The femoral artery was checked again and it still had a 2+ pulse. Sutures were secured. Hemostasis was noted. The retroperitoneum was irrigated. Again, hemostasis was noted. A JP drain was placed subfascially through a right lower quadrant stab incision and secured to the skin with 2-0 nylon. The fascia was then closed in 1 layer using looped #1 PDS. The subcutaneous tissue was closed with 3-0 Vicryl and the skin was closed with staples. A sterile dressing was applied and the patient was extubated and transported to the recovery room in stable condition, having tolerated the procedure well.

ESTIMATED BLOOD LOSS: Less than 100 cc

Needle, sponge, and instrument counts correct.

SPECIMENS: Transplanted kidney

The patient received 250 cc of 5% albumin and 100 cc of normal saline.

Answer Sheet

Directions: Be sure to enter all medical record codes in the manner provided in the sample below, paying special attention to the decimal placement for each code. The codes must be typed on the answer sheet in the boxes provided on the computer screen using the keyboard. A decimal point (.) has been provided as a guide for entering each ICD-9-CM code. **You will lose credit if the digits of the codes are correct, but the decimal point has been incorrectly placed.**

CASE 12 DIAGNOSES   **ICD-9-CM**

DX1				.		
DX2				.		
DX3				.		
DX4				.		

CASE 12 PROCEDURES   **CPT/HCPCS**

PR1					
PR2					
PR3					
PR4					
PR5					
PR6					

CASE STUDY 13

*Please code for the services of the physician
and the office.*

Practice Exam 3   CASE 13

Neurodiagnostic Laboratory

PATIENT HISTORY: The patient is a 39-year-old woman sent for evaluation of right wrist pain. The patient is 26 weeks pregnant and peripheral edema is thought to play a role here. The patient denies any significant neck pain with radiation. She states she gets tingling and numbness of the digits intermittently, often occurring with gripping activities. She often wakes up in the morning with the thumb unable to straighten out. On PE, she had intact and symmetrical DTRs at the biceps, triceps, and finger flexors. Tone is normal. Muscle bulk is intact. The DTRs of the patella are brisk. There is no ankle clonus and tone is normal.

Motor Nerve Conduction

Nerve and Site	Latency 1	Amplitude	Segment Name	Distance	Conduction Velocity	Corrected Velocity
Median nerve R						
Wrist	4.7 ms	4.570 mV		80 mm	m/s	m/s
Elbow	8.9 ms	3.880 mV	Wrist-elbow	210 mm	50 m/s	m/s
Ulnar nerve R						
Wrist	3.2 ms	13.48 mV		80 mm	m/s	m/s
Below elbow	6.5 ms	11.81 mV	Wrist-below elbow	195 mm	59 m/s	m/s
Mid-arm	8.1 ms	11.46 mV	Below elbow—Mid-arm	80 mm	56 m/s	m/s

Sensory Nerve Conduction

Nerve and Site	Peak Latency	Amplitude	Segment	Onset Latency	Distance	Conduction Velocity	Corrected Velocity
Median nerve R							
Wrist (14 cm)	4.2 ms	40.47 uV	Index-wrist 14 cm	3.3 ms	140 mm	m/s	m/s
Ulnar Nerve R							
Wrist 14 cm	3.6 ms	47.87 uV	Digit V—Wrist 14 cm	2.7 ms	140 mm	m/s	m/s
Median/Ulnar Palmer R							
Palm (Med)	2.6 ms	19.22 uV	Wrist 8 cm—Palm (Med)	2.1 ms	100 mm	m/s	m/s
Palm (Uln)	1.9 ms	30.021 uV	Wrist 8 cm—Palm (Uln)	1.4 ms	100 mm	m/s	m/s

Needle EMG Data

		Insertional	Spontaneous Activity			Motor Unit Description				Recruitment			
			Fibs	+ Wave	Fasucs	Poly	Amp 1st MU	MUP Dur	MUP Config	Frequency	Max Pattern	Max Effort	Rec Ratio
1st Dorsal Interossei	R		None	None	None	None	Norm	Norm	Norm	Norm	Full	Full	Normal
Abd Pollicis Brevis (C8T1)	R		None	None	None	None	2k	Norm	Norm	Norm	Red	Full	Mild Inc.
Biceps Brachii (C56)			None	None	None	None	Norm	Norm	Norm	Norm	Full	Full	Normal
Triceps (C78)			None	None	None	None	Norm	Norm	Norm	Norm	Full	Full	Normal
Pronator Teres(C67)			None	None	None	None	Norm	Norm	Norm	Norm	Full	Full	Normal

CONCLUSION:

ABNORMAL EXAMINATION: There is evidence of carpal tunnel syndrome on the right. This is approaching moderate severity with mild axonal degeneration present. There is no evidence of an ulnar neuropathy at the wrist or across the elbow. There is no evidence of an acute or significant chronic left C5-T1 or right C8-T1 radiculopathy.

CLINICAL NOTE: The patient tolerated this electrodiagnostic examination quite well overall.

Answer Sheet

Directions: Be sure to enter all medical record codes in the manner provided in the sample below, paying special attention to the decimal placement for each code. The codes must be typed on the answer sheet in the boxes provided on the computer screen using the keyboard. A decimal point (.) has been provided as a guide for entering each ICD-9-CM code. **You will lose credit if the digits of the codes are correct, but the decimal point has been incorrectly placed.**

CASE 13 DIAGNOSES   **ICD-9-CM**

DX1				.		
DX2				.		
DX3				.		
DX4				.		

CASE 13 PROCEDURES   **CPT/HCPCS**

PR1					
PR2					
PR3					
PR4					
PR5					
PR6					

CASE STUDY 14

Please code for the services of the physician.

Practice Exam 3   CASE 14

REASON FOR VISIT: Left leg pain

HISTORY OF PRESENT ILLNESS: This is an 80-year-old diabetic resident at Nursing Manor. Patient has had this open wound in her left lower leg being dressed by nursing home staff twice a week. It has continued to get smaller, although for the past 5 days, she started having pain in the left leg that will start at the open wound and shoot all the way up to her hip. She has no fever or chills. Blood sugars are checking "normal" running around 114–120.

PHYSICAL EXAMINATION: Weight: 202, blood pressure: 130/58

This is an 80-year-old in no acute distress.

EXTREMITIES: Examination of her left leg shows no new swelling. There is some mild erythema around the open wound with some yellow exudate.

IMPRESSION:

1. Cellulitis, left leg
2. Diabetic peripheral vascular disease

PLAN: The patient was given 1 g of Rocephin IV push today in the office. Continue the dressings per Nursing Manor staff nurses. She may continue her pain medicine as needed. Recheck as needed.

HISTORY: Expanded problem

EXAMINATION: Expanded problem

MEDICAL DECISION-MAKING: Moderate

Answer Sheet

Directions: Be sure to enter all medical record codes in the manner provided in the sample below, paying special attention to the decimal placement for each code. The codes must be typed on the answer sheet in the boxes provided on the computer screen using the keyboard. A decimal point (.) has been provided as a guide for entering each ICD-9-CM code. **You will lose credit if the digits of the codes are correct, but the decimal point has been incorrectly placed.**

CASE 14 DIAGNOSES   **ICD-9-CM**

DX1				.	
DX2				.	
DX3				.	
DX4				.	

CASE 14 PROCEDURES   **CPT/HCPCS**

PR1					
PR2					
PR3					
PR4					
PR5					
PR6					

CASE STUDY 15

Please code for the services of the physician.

Practice Exam 3

CASE 15

In-Office Chemotherapy Administration

The patient is a 73-year-old woman who arrives today for her scheduled chemotherapy treatment. All injections are sequential. She is being treated for serious papillary ovarian cancer with metastasis to the lungs.

Treatment today:

Carboplatin infusion, 50 mg
    Start time 1:30 PM, End time 2:05 PM

Paclitaxel infusion, 25 mg
    Start time 2:06 PM, End time 3:10 PM

Ondansetron infusion, 1 mg
    Start time 3:12 PM, End time 3:32 PM

Answer Sheet

Directions: Be sure to enter all medical record codes in the manner provided in the sample below, paying special attention to the decimal placement for each code. The codes must be typed on the answer sheet in the boxes provided on the computer screen using the keyboard. A decimal point (.) has been provided as a guide for entering each ICD-9-CM code. **You will lose credit if the digits of the codes are correct, but the decimal point has been incorrectly placed.**

CASE 15 DIAGNOSES   **ICD-9-CM**

					.		
DX1					.		
DX2					.		
DX3					.		
DX4					.		

CASE 15 PROCEDURES   **CPT/HCPCS**

PR1					
PR2					
PR3					
PR4					
PR5					
PR6					

CASE STUDY 16

Please code for the services of the surgeon.

Practice Exam 3   CASE 16

PREOPERATIVE DIAGNOSES: Status post liver transplant secondary to biliary atresia, and dental caries

POSTOPERATIVE DIAGNOSES: Status post liver transplant secondary to biliary atresia, and dental caries

OPERATION: Primary teeth extractions

INDICATIONS: Multiple dental caries in a non-English-speaking boy age 4 years, 10 months. Because of his transplant status, it was thought that his care would best be provided under general anesthesia. Medicaid will pay for extraction.

FINDINGS: Intact primary dentition is present. There are caries in the teeth in the following manner: tooth #K—occlusal buccal, tooth #S—buccal occlusal distal mesial, tooth #T—occlusal buccal. Decalcification is noted on the facial of tooth #C, tooth #D and tooth #H. Gingival health is fair throughout the mouth. Minimal plaque is noted on all teeth. Tooth #K, #S and #T had carious pulpal exposures and/or hyperemic pulpal tissue.

PROCEDURE: The patient was brought to the operating room in a sedated state. Nasotracheal intubation was completed and a moist throat pack was placed. A total of 36 mg 2% lidocaine with 18 mcg of epinephrine was deposited adjacent to tooth #K, tooth #S, and tooth #T in preparation for extraction. All three teeth were extracted intact using forceps in a routine manner. Sockets were curetted. Instat was placed. The oral cavity was rinsed and suctioned, and the throat pack was removed. The patient was then extubated and transferred to the recovery room in stable, sedated condition.

Answer Sheet

Directions: Be sure to enter all medical record codes in the manner provided in the sample below, paying special attention to the decimal placement for each code. The codes must be typed on the answer sheet in the boxes provided on the computer screen using the keyboard. A decimal point (.) has been provided as a guide for entering each ICD-9-CM code. **You will lose credit if the digits of the codes are correct, but the decimal point has been incorrectly placed.**

CASE 16 DIAGNOSES   **ICD-9-CM**

					.		
DX1					.		
DX2					.		
DX3					.		
DX4					.		

CASE 16 PROCEDURES   **CPT/HCPCS**

PR1					
PR2					
PR3					
PR4					
PR5					
PR6					

Answer Key

Practice Answers

1. B   The integrated health record is arranged in strict chronological order with different types of information and sources of information mixed together according to the data on the entries. Physicians' offices often use this format (LaTour and Eichenwald Maki, 186).

2. B   The condition listed in this question is the only one that is not a complication of labor and delivery. All of the others listed here are complications (according to the *ICD-9-CM Codebook*) and are to be coded as such (Hazelwood and Venable, 209).

3. C   Methicillin-resistant staphylococcus aureus is considered as a major source of hospital-acquired infections.

4. A   This is one of the prion diseases.

5. B   Synthroid is given to patients to augment or replace small levels of thyroid hormone, thyroxine.

6. C   Klebsiella is the only gram-negative organism listed; all others are gram-positive (Hazelwood and Venable, 71).

7. B   The codes in the preventive medicine services category of CPT are used to report the preventive medicine E/M of infants, children, adolescents, and adults. They are assigned based on the patient's age (Kuehn, 70).

8. D   The physician should be queried when information is not documented and a more specific code could be assigned.

9. B   Clinical data is the most common type of health information and it documents the signs, symptoms, diagnoses, impressions, treatments, and outcomes of the care process (LaTour and Eichenwald Maki, 89).

10. C   Pathology reports are required for cases in which a surgical specimen is removed or expelled during a procedure. Specimens are examined both microscopically and macroscopically (LaTour and Eichenwald Maki, 200).

11. B   A radiologist's findings may be used to clarify an outpatient's diagnosis or reason for services. Based on the fact that the radiologist is a physician, a coder can do a diagnosis from the x-ray (Schraffenberger, 256).

12. A   Code V30.00 also requires the use of an "Outcome of Delivery" code; An *M code* is used secondarily to provide the morphology for a neoplasm code and follows the code for the neoplasm; and *E codes* follow the trauma, disease, or injury code and provides detail as to how the situation happened (Hazelwood and Venable, 38–39).

13. D   A fetal death refers to the death of a fetus of a particular weight or gestation, frequently 500 g or more or 22 or more completed weeks of gestation, though the weight and week gestation may vary from state to state (Brodnik, 274).

14. C   In this situation, the patient had drowsiness due to an intentional overdose of a drug which classifies it as a "poisoning" using the Suicide Attempt column of the Table of External Causes (Hazelwood and Venable, 265–266).

15. A   In this situation, the patient had an accidental overdose of a drug which classifies it as a poisoning and utilizes the "accident" column of the External Cause Table (Hazelwood and Venable, 265–266).

16. C   The term "missed abortion" refers to fetal death that occurs prior to the completion of 22 weeks of gestation (Brown, 300).

17. C   A diagnosis of elevated blood pressure reading, without a diagnosis of hypertension is assigned code 796.2. The physician must have specifically documented a diagnosis of elevated blood pressure (Brown, 350).

18. B   Infants born to RH-negative mothers often develop hemolytic disease owing to fetal-maternal blood group incompatibility. These conditions are classified to Category 773, hemolytic disease of fetus or newborn, due to isoimmunization (Brown, 317).

19. A   The patient had a second-degree laceration (not a third-degree laceration) and the outcome of delivery code is V27.0, not V27.9 which is for unspecified outcome of delivery (Brown, 282).

20. A   In ICD-9-CM, the coding guidelines for late effects is to code the residual condition (monoplegia) of the late effect first, followed by the cause of the late effect (poliomyelitis) (Hazelwood and Venable, 55).

21. C   In some cases symptoms are coded as additional diagnoses when they "represent important problems in medical care." With this question, it would be important to code the coma since it impacts the metastasis to the brain (Hazelwood and Venable, 61).

22. A   When a patient seeks health care for the purpose of contraceptive sterilization, code V25.2 is assigned as the principal diagnosis (Brown, 283).

23. C   (Kuehn, 16.)

24. A   Emergency Department E/M services require all three components to be met or exceeded. The service provided—the ED physician only did a detailed history and a detailed exam—only meets level 99284. The spinal puncture is diagnostic and therefore, 62270 (Kuehn, 62–63).

25. D   Morselized bone is bone that has been crushed to conform to the area receiving the graft. You can read about spine surgery in *The Lumbar Spine* by Harry N. Herkowitz, 74–76 (Kuehn, 124).

26. C   (*CPT Professional Edition,* 108) (*Dorland's Medical Dictionary*—shoulder blade; saucerization)

27. D   Destruction codes are used because the physician curettes the lesions, which is included as a method of destruction. In addition, the lesions are actinic keratoses, which are listed as a form of premalignant lesions that are normally destroyed using this method (Kuehn, 115).

28. A   An indirect laryngoscopy uses a mirror to visualize the larynx. A direct laryngoscopy would use an endoscope. The diagnostic laryngoscopy is included in the endoscopy for removal of the foreign body (Kuehn, 134).

29. A   The coding notes before code 64490 state that bilateral injections should be coded using a –50 modifier and that injections on the T12–L1 level are coded with 64493 (*CPT Professional Edition,* 314).

30. C   The *Coder Desk Reference* shows the following for code 33814: "The physician gains access to the mediastinum through an incision through the sternum (median sternotomy). The physician places cardiopulmonary bypass catheters through incisions in the low inferior vena cava, the superior vena cava, and high aorta or femoral artery. The physician stops the heart by infusing cardioplegia solution into the coronary circulation. The physician cross-clamps the aorta, places sump suction in the left atrium to obtain a bloodless surgical field. The physician exposes the aortopulmonary septal defect by cutting through the ascending aorta or main pulmonary artery. The physician closes the defect with a Dacron fabric patch, closes the aortic or pulmonary arterial incision, takes the patient off cardiopulmonary bypass, closes the remaining surgical incisions and dresses the sternal wound. The physician may leave chest tubes and/or a mediastinal drainage tube in place following the procedure." (Ingenix, 314). This is the procedure performed in this question.

31. C   Code 16025 describes the specific work associated with débridement of a burn wound and wound dressing (*CPT Assistant,* August 1997, 08(7), 6–7).

32. B   This colonography service is new in the CPT category I codes for 2010. Code 74262 correctly describes the service listed in this question (*CPT Changes 2010—An Insider's View,* 145).

33. C   Tests that are ordered together and performed together that are listed together as a panel must be billed as a panel. If all the tests listed in a panel are not performed, they must be billed individually. In this case, all of the tests listed in the electrolyte panel were performed and must be coded together as 80051 (Kuehn, 223).

34. C   The psychotherapy codes are assigned based on time. Each time-based code has an option to include minimal E/M services, such as prescription drug management (Kuehn, 241).

35. B   The allergist provides single-dose vials as indicated in CPT code 95144 (Kuehn, 251–252).

36. B   This service requires a 99283 Emergency Department code (due to expanded problem focused history), the code for the rabies immune globulin and the administration and rabies vaccine and the vaccine administration (Kuehn, 239).

37. B   This question says that the imaging was performed by the radiologist. Therefore, code 10022 cannot be correct because it includes imaging. In addition, the question does not state that the needle biopsy was a fine needle biopsy, which is different. The biopsy is not stated as a wedge biopsy and therefore code 47100 is incorrect. Because code 47000 describes the procedure, the unlisted code of 47399 would not be used (*CPT Assistant,* Fall 1993, 03(3), 11–20).

38. B   The islet cells are transplanted through an incision, therefore the procedure is open (*CPT Assistant* June 2007, 17(6), 7–9).

39. C   The Category III code describes all of the work necessary to insert the spinous process distraction device, the work described in this question (*CPT Assistant* July 2007, Volume 17(7), 6–10).

40. C   Each unit of the drug is worth 250 mg. 600 mg is more than 2 units and less than 3 units. Therefore, 3 units are reported (Kuehn, 273).

41. B   The combination code of complex cystometrogram and voiding pressure studies is the only code required. This procedure would be correctly coded by including the –26 modifier to describe the urologist's professional services (Kuehn, 164).

42. C   Dr. Smith receives 80% of the Medicare allowed amount which is $160. Dr. Jones receives nothing from CMS because he does not accept assignment. The patient receives the benefits.

43. C   Dr. Smith will receive the entire $200 minus $160 from CMS and the remaining 20% or $40 from the patient. Dr. Jones will receive $218.50 from the patient. This amount is the most he can charge under CMS' limiting charge rule. This figure is derived by determining the non-PAR allowed charge which is 95% of the PAR amount—in this case, that would be $190. The limiting charge = 115% of that amount or $218.50.

44. C   Medicare typically doesn't cover preventive medicine but a new benefit was provided in The Medicare Prescription Drug, Improvement, and Modernization Act of 2003 that provides one preventive physical examination, or the "Welcome to Medicare Physical," for new Medicare Part B enrollees within the first 12 months of entitlement (Kuehn, 69).

45. A   When referencing Column 1 and Column 2 NCCI edits, the modifier would be applied to the code in Column 2 (Kuehn, 306–308).

46. C   The conversion factor is the across-the-board multiplier for the RBRVS system. The conversion factor is a constant that applies to the entire RVU. The conversion factor is the government's most direct control on Medicare payments to physicians. CMS raises or lowers the conversion factor to raise or lower physician payments (Casto and Layman, 160).

47. A   A formulary for drugs, a copayment and benefit limitations are all provisions for cost-sharing between the beneficiary and the insurance company. A benefit is what is provided to the patient (Casto and Layman, 52–54).

48. A   A diagnosis distribution report will show all of the ICD-9-CM codes used during the selected time period and will allow the office manager to identify issues such as missing digits, use of nonspecific codes, and inappropriate to setting usage (Kuehn, 315).

49. B   The characteristics of data quality are listed as follows: accuracy, accessibility, comprehensives, consistency, currency, definition, granularity, integrity, precision, relevancy, and timeliness. Analysis is not listed as a characteristic (Abdelhak, 144).

50. C   Modifier AI is now required for patients covered by Medicare when reporting Initial Hospital Service codes and this modifier is missing from the code (Kuehn, 58).

51. C   A line graph is often used to display time trends. The *x*-axis shows a unit of time and the *y*-axis measures the value of the variable being plotted (LaTour and Eichenwald Maki, 424–426).

52. C   Computer-assisted coding is not a magic bullet. It cannot address the major obstacle facing today's human coder: the lack of accurate, complete clinical documentation (LaTour and Eichenwald Maki, 401).

53. C   Data mapping describes the connections or paths between classifications and vocabularies. Data mining refers to the process of extracting information from a database and then filtering discrete, structured data. Redundancy is the process by which data entered into one server is simultaneously entered into a second server (LaTour and Eichenwald Maki, 250, 962).

54. D   AHIMA defines computer-assisted coding (CAC) as the use of computer software that automatically generates a set of medical codes for review validation, and use based upon the documentation provided by the various providers of healthcare (LaTour and Eichenwald Maki, 400).

55. D   An advance directive is a legal, written document that specifies patient preferences regarding future health care or specifies another person to make medical decisions in the event the patient has an incurable, or irreversible condition and is unable to communicate his or her wishes (Abdelhak, 13).

56. C   The HIPAA Privacy and Security Rules apply to PHI used or disclosed by covered entities. Covered entities are healthcare providers, healthcare clearinghouses, and health plans that conduct the financial and administrative transactions described in the Transaction and Code Sets Rule (TCS). If an individual provider or an organization does not fit within the definitions of a healthcare provider, clearinghouse, or health plan, the rules do not apply (Roach, 141).

57. A   HIM professionals must resist the temptation to overlook inadequate documentation and report codes without appropriate clinical foundation within the record just to speed up claims processing, meet a business requirement, or obtain additional reimbursement (Hazelwood and Venable, 328).

58. B   The HIPAA "minimum necessary" principle/standard has to be applied to determining employee access to PHI (Brodnick, 245).

59. B   HIPAA defers to state laws on matters concerning minors; therefore, consult state laws regarding the rules for appropriate authorization (Brodnick, 107).

60. D   Regardless of whether the patient is an adult or a minor, the law allows a presumption of consent during an emergency situation (Brodnick, 99).

CASE 1 DIAGNOSES   ICD-9-CM

DX1 Type I diabetes mellitus with ketoacidosis	2	5	0	.	1	3
DX2 Reactive airway disease	4	9	3	.	9	2
DX3				.		
DX4				.		

CASE 1 PROCEDURES   CPT/HCPCS

PR1 Subsequent inpatient pediatric critical care	9	9	4	7	6
PR2					
PR3					
PR4					
PR5					
PR6					

CASE 2 DIAGNOSES   ICD-9-CM

DX1 Hodgkins, nodular sclerosis	2	0	1	.	5	0
DX2				.		
DX3				.		
DX4				.		

CASE 2 PROCEDURES   CPT/HCPCS

PR1 Bone marrow biopsy, needle	3	8	2	2	1
PR2					
PR3					
PR4					
PR5					
PR6					

CASE 3 DIAGNOSES

ICD-9-CM

DX1 Temporal lobe epilepsy	3	4	5	.	4	0
DX2				.		
DX3				.		
DX4				.		

CASE 3 PROCEDURES

CPT/HCPCS

PR1 Office or other outpatient consultation	9	9	2	4	5
PR2 Electroencephalogram, awake and asleep	9	5	8	1	9
PR3					
PR4					
PR5					
PR6					

CASE 4 DIAGNOSES

ICD-9-CM

DX1 Congenital defect of nasal sidewall	7	4	8	.	1	
DX2				.		
DX3				.		
DX4				.		

CASE 4 PROCEDURES

CPT/HCPCS

PR1 Full-thickness graft, 20 sq cm or less	1	5	2	6	0
PR2 Graft, ear cartilage, autogenous to nose or ear	2	1	2	3	5
PR3					
PR4					
PR5					
PR6					

CASE 5 DIAGNOSES   ICD-9-CM

DX1 ADHD	3	1	4	.	0	1
DX2 Reactive adjustment disorder with anxiety	3	0	9	.	2	4
DX3				.		
DX4				.		

CASE 5 PROCEDURES   CPT/HCPCS

PR1 Individual psychotherapy, 45 to 50 minutes, with medical E/M service	9	0	8	0	7
PR2					
PR3					
PR4					
PR5					
PR6					

CASE 6 DIAGNOSES   **ICD-9-CM**

DX1 Labral tear	8	4	3	.	8	
DX2				.		
DX3				.		
DX4				.		

CASE 6 PROCEDURES   **CPT/HCPCS**

PR1 Unlisted procedure, arthroscopy	2	9	9	9	9
PR2					
PR3					
PR4					
PR5					
PR6					

CASE 7 DIAGNOSES   **ICD-9-CM**

DX1 Generalized abdominal pain	7	8	9	.	0	7
DX2				.		
DX3				.		
DX4				.		

CASE 7 PROCEDURES   **CPT/HCPCS**

PR1 Colonoscopy, flexible with biopsy, single or multiple	4	5	3	8	0
PR2 EGD with biopsy, single or multiple	4	3	2	3	9
PR3					
PR4					
PR5					
PR6					

CASE 8 DIAGNOSES   **ICD-9-CM**

DX1 Iron deficiency anemia	2	8	0	.	9	
DX2 Renal hypertension	4	0	3	.	9	0
DX3 Chronic kidney disease, stage III	5	8	5	.	3	
DX4 Type II diabetes	2	5	0	.	0	0

CASE 8 PROCEDURES   **CPT/HCPCS**

PR1 IV, initial, up to 1 hour	9	6	3	6	5
PR2 IV, each additional hour	9	6	3	6	6
PR3 IV, each additional hour	9	6	3	6	6
PR4 IV push	9	6	3	7	4
PR5 Diphenhydramine HCl, up to 50 mg	J	1	2	0	0
PR6 Famotidine, 20 mg	S	0	0	2	8

Practice Exam 1 Answers

1. A   For outpatient services (as is the case in this example) the coder may use documentation provided by a pathologist. Therefore, the coder should code the lesion as a basal cell carcinoma.

2. D   Preventive medicine services category codes are assigned based on the age of the patient (Kuehn, 68–70).

3. C   The total size of a removed lesion, including margins, is needed for accurate coding. This information is best provided in the operative report. The pathology report typically provides the specimen size rather than the size of the excised lesion. Because the specimen tends to shrink, this is not an accurate measurement (Kuehn, 108).

4. B   Protonix is used to treat patients with erosive esophagitis associated with GERD. It decreases the accumulation of acid in the stomach. More information on Protonix is available at http://www.drugs.com/protonix.html.

5. C   Haldol is used to treat symptoms of schizophrenia. More information on Haldol is available at http://www.drugs.com/cdi/haldol.html.

6. D   Status asthmaticus is an acute asthmatic attack in which the degree of bronchial obstruction is not relieved by usual treatments such as epinephrine or aminophylline. A patient in status asthmaticus fails to respond to therapy (Schraffenberger, 173). Only a physician can diagnose status asthmaticus. If a coder suspects the condition based on the symptoms documented in the record, the coder should query the physician about the documentation for status asthmaticus.

7. C   A serous papillary adenocarcinoma usually originates in the ovary.

8. A   Hypokalemia is defined as decreased levels of potassium in the blood.

9. B   Medication records are maintained for all patients and include medications given, time, form of administration, dosage, and strength. The records are updated when the patient is given the medication. Nursing personnel complete the medication records (LaTour and Eichenwald Maki, 199).

10. B   The *ICD-9-CM Official Guidelines for Coding and Reporting,* Section IV. Diagnostic Coding and Reporting Guidelines for Outpatient Services indicate that when a physician qualifies a diagnostic statement as "rule out", the condition qualified in that statement should not be coded as if it existed. Rather, the condition should be coded to the highest level of certainty, such as the signs and symptoms the patient exhibits (Kuehn, 29–31).

11. C   A series of terms in parentheses, called nonessential modifiers, sometimes directly follows a main term or subterm (Hazelwood and Venable, 14).

12. B   A section mark symbol precedes codes in the Tabular List of both diseases and procedures. It indicates the presence of a footnote at the bottom of the page or references an instructional note located earlier in the section (Hazelwood and Venable, 26).

13. A   Slanted, or italicized, brackets are found only in the Alphabetic Index and enclose a code number that must be used in conjunction with a code immediately preceding it (Hazelwood and Venable, 25).

14. D   When coding late effects, the residual condition or nature of the late effect is sequenced first, followed by the cause of the late effect (Hazelwood and Venable, 51).

15. B   The other organisms listed are either viruses or fungi. *Staphylococcus aureus* is the only bacteria in this list (Hazelwood and Venable, 68).

16. B   In ICD-9-CM, an elderly primigravida is defined as a woman who gives birth to her first child after age 35 (Brown, 274).

17. D   According to the National Center for Health Statistics and the American College of Obstetricians and Gynecologists, Early Onset of Delivery should be assigned for an abortion resulting in a liveborn infant. In addition to code 644.21, a code for the outcome of delivery (V27) may be assigned (Hazelwood and Venable, 203).

18. B   Category 650, Normal delivery, is assigned when all of the following criteria are met: a) delivery of a full-term, single, healthy liveborn infant; b) delivery without prenatal or postpartum complications; or c) cephalic or occipital presentation with spontaneous, vaginal delivery requiring minimal or no assistance, with or without episiotomy, without fetal manipulation or instrumentation (Hazelwood and Venable, 206).

19. A   The perinatal, or newborn, period is defined as beginning before birth and lasting through 28 days after birth. There is also an inclusion note at the beginning of Chapter 15 reminding the coder of this definition (Hazelwood and Venable, 219).

20. C   Category 645, Late pregnancy, is used to demonstrate that a woman is past 40 weeks' gestation (Hazelwood and Venable, 207).

21. D   A common congenital cardiac defect, ventricular septal defect, is defined as an abnormal communication or opening in the ventricular septum that allows the blood to shunt from the left ventricle to the right ventricle (Hazelwood and Venable, 217–218).

22. C   Code 775.0, Syndrome of "infant of a diabetic mother," should be assigned when the newborn infant of a diabetic mother or gestational diabetic mother manifests features of this condition (Hazelwood and Venable, 105).

23. B   In ICD-9-CM, Category V22 includes codes for supervision of a normal pregnancy. Generally, code V22.0 is for supervision of normal first pregnancy (Hazelwood and Venable, 35).

24. B   In ICD-9-CM, Category 651, Multiple Gestation, has fourth digit subcategories that indicate the number of fetuses and fifth digit subcategories denoting the current episode of care (Hazelwood and Venable, 208).

25. B   Option B defines when time can be used to select the E/M code (Kuehn, 52).

26. C   See Coding Guidelines codes 33202–33249 (*CPT Professional Edition,* 164).

27. B   This question is the classic description of two surgeons performing one procedure (Kuehn, 281–282).

28. C   Unlisted codes are to be used when there is no other code within CPT that correctly describes the service (*CPT Professional Edition,* 8, 53).

29. B   PTCAs are coded to 92982 when performed on a single coronary vessel (*CPT Professional Edition,* 456).

30. B   The only modifier in the list that is eligible for use with an E/M code is the –32 modifier (Kuehn, 62).

31. D   *CPT Professional Edition,* index page 755 instructs the coder to see pages 73–74 for the TRAM procedure. In this example, the coder should recognize that Transverse Rectus Abdominis Myocutaneous is the meaning of the abbreviation TRAM.

32. C   The documentation includes that the bone fragments pierced the dura, therefore the two codes describing extradural procedures are not appropriate. Cranioplasty is not described in the documentation. Code 62010 for the elevation of the depressed skull fracture with repair of dura and/or débridement of brain describes the performed procedures.

33. D   The coder should always reference the codes found in the Tabular Index before code assignment (Kuehn, 19–20).

34. B   This is the definition of the codes used to describe admission and discharge on the same calendar date (*CPT Professional Edition,* 15) (Kuehn, 59).

35. D   Secondary procedures are those that are performed following previous surgery. Option D, code 66172, describes that this surgery is done following a previous ocular surgery (Kuehn, 188).

36. C   This question clearly defines a domiciliary (Kuehn, 65–66).

37. C   A heart system transplant is coded with a category III code because no category I code is available.

38. C   Documentation does not state the structures where the foreign body was found, only that it was driven deep into the plantar surface of the foot, therefore, the appropriate code is 28192.

39. A   (Casto and Layman, 240.)

40. A   Claims submission is the process of submitting claims data to third-party payers (Kuehn, 309–310).

41. A   The CMS-1500 form is the standard billing document used for physician claims submitted on paper for Medicare Part B reimbursement. Providers also use this form for paper claims submitted to many private health insurance companies and Medicaid agencies (Kuehn, 309).

42. C   A provider that participates with an insurance plan (including Medicare) and has a contractual arrangement with the plan to provide care and bill the plan directly for the services provided is known as a participating provider or PAR (Kuehn, 297).

43. D   Deductible is the amount of cost, usually annual, that the policyholder must incur (and pay) before the insurance plan will assume liability for remaining covered expenses (AHIMA, 84).

44. A   The RBRVS system is the federal government's payment system for physicians. It is a system of classifying health services based on the cost of furnishing physicians' services in different settings, the skill and training levels required to perform the services, and the time and risk involved (Casto and Layman, 157).

45. B   (Schraffenberger, 60.)

46. C   The Remittance Advice reports claim rejections, denials, and payments to the practice (Casto and Layman, 212, 254) (Kuehn, 337–338).

47. D   Each time a questionable service is provided, an ABN must be provided (Kuehn, 303).

48. B   Linking informs the payer which diagnosis is associated with each procedure on the claim (Kuehn, 305).

49. D   The Medicare Prescription Drug, Improvement, and Modernization Act was signed in 2003. Section 503 of this bill includes wording stating that beginning in 2005, ICD-9-CM diagnosis and procedure codes could be issued to be effective twice a year—April 1 and October 1 (Hazelwood and Venable, 3).

50. B   When the coder compares the procedure description to the diagnosis description, there is a difference between the location of the foreign body; therefore, the diagnosis was not correctly linked to the procedure.

51. C   Allowing the physician to select the codes for an audit will not ensure a representative sample (Kuehn, 356).

52. A   None of the claims in the list are correct; therefore, the problem is CPT coding accuracy. A three-level cervical laminectomy is coded as 63045, 63048, 63048 (Kuehn, 182–183).

53. A   This production report does not contain any entries for new patient E/M codes. It is highly unlikely that all patients that have not been seen previously were seen at the request of another healthcare provider. Therefore, the physician may require education on the definition of new patient visits (Kuehn, 43).

54. C   Electronic spreadsheets can be used to facilitate data collection and analysis. The advantage of spreadsheets is that charts and graphs can be formulated as the data are being analyzed.

55. A Encryption is the process of transforming text into an unintelligible string of characters that can be transmitted via communications media with a high degree of security and then decrypted when it reaches a secure destination (LaTour and Eichenwald Maki, 78).

56. A AHIMA's Code of Ethics are ethical principles that are based on the core values of AHIMA. "Coding an intentionally inappropriate level of service" violates "IV—Refuse to participate in or conceal unethical practices or procedures" of AHIMA's Code of Ethics (AHIMA HOD 2008) (Hazelwood and Venable, 313–317).

57. A The Centers for Medicare and Medicaid Services (CMS) and the National Center for Health Statistics (NCHS) provide the official guidelines for coding and reporting using ICD-9-CM. These guides have been approved by the four organizations that make up the Cooperating Parities for the ICD-9-CM: The American Hospital Association, AHIMA, CMS, and NCHS (Hazelwood and Venable, 327).

58. B When offenses are discovered, they should be investigated and corrective measures undertaken. Physician practices should develop indicators that would signal a problem. Corrective action may include refunding overpayments from a third-party payer or even self-reporting to the government (Hazelwood and Venable, 301).

59. C Developing, coordinating, and participating in coding training programs falls under the area of monitoring compliance efforts of the practice, whereas the other answers are actual risk areas identified by the OIG (Hazelwood and Venable, 300).

60. C Medicare defines "abuse" as involving billing practices that are inconsistent with generally acceptable fiscal policies. This usually results from inadvertent coding or billing mistakes and is not considered fraudulent (Hazelwood and Venable, 299).

CASE 1 DIAGNOSES   ICD-9-CM

DX1 Pneumonia	4	8	6	.		
DX2 Tobacco use disorder	3	0	5	.	1	
DX3				.		
DX4				.		

CASE 1 PROCEDURES   CPT/HCPCS

PR1 Office and other outpatient E/M, new	9	9	2	0	4
PR2 IV push	9	6	3	7	4
PR3 Levofloxacin (Levaquin) 250 mg	J	1	9	5	6
PR4 Levofloxacin (Levaquin) 250 mg	J	1	9	5	6
PR5					
PR6					

CASE 2 DIAGNOSES   **ICD-9-CM**

DX1 Respiratory failure	5	1	8	.	8	1
DX2 Pulmonary contusion	8	6	1	.	2	1
DX3 *Haemophilus influenzae*	0	4	1	.	5	
DX4				.		

CASE 2 PROCEDURES   **CPT/HCPCS**

PR1 Critical care, 1st hour	9	9	2	9	1
PR2					
PR3					
PR4					
PR5					
PR6					

CASE 3 DIAGNOSES   **ICD-9-CM**

DX1 Diarrhea	7	8	7	.	9	1
DX2 Nausea	7	8	7	.	0	2
DX3 Abrasions	9	1	3	.	0	
DX4				.		

CASE 3 PROCEDURES   **CPT/HCPCS**

PR1 Office and other outpatient E/M, establish	9	9	2	1	4
PR2 Immunization administration, 1st vaccine	9	0	4	7	1
PR3 Tetanus and diphtheria toxoid vaccine	9	0	7	1	8
PR4					
PR5					
PR6					

CASE 4 DIAGNOSES   **ICD-9-CM**

DX1 Type I diabetes mellitus	2	5	0	.	1	3
DX2 Constipation	5	6	4	.	0	0
DX3				.		
DX4				.		

CASE 4 PROCEDURES   **CPT/HCPCS**

PR1 Inpatient consultation	9	9	2	5	5
PR2					
PR3					
PR4					
PR5					
PR6					

CASE 5 DIAGNOSES   ICD-9-CM

				.		
DX1 Complication following AB	6	3	9	.	8	
DX2 Urinary tract infection	5	9	9	.	0	
DX3				.		
DX4				.		

CASE 5 PROCEDURES   CPT/HCPCS

PR1 Emergency department E/M	9	9	2	8	4
PR2					
PR3					
PR4					
PR5					
PR6					

CASE 6 DIAGNOSES　　　　　　　　　　　　　　　**ICD-9-CM**

DX1 Irregular heartbeat (bigeminy)	4	2	7	.	8	9
DX2				.		
DX3				.		
DX4				.		

CASE 6 PROCEDURES　　　　　　　　　　　　　　　**CPT/HCPCS**

PR1 Outpatient consultation	9	9	2	4	2
PR2 Echocardiography, 2D	9	3	3	0	7
PR3					
PR4					
PR5					
PR6					

CASE 7 DIAGNOSES   **ICD-9-CM**

DX1 Hashimoto's thyroiditis	2	4	5	.	2	
DX2				.		
DX3				.		
DX4				.		

CASE 7 PROCEDURES   **CPT/HCPCS**

PR1 Total thyroid lobectomy, unilateral; with or without isthmusectomy	6	0	2	2	0
PR2					
PR3					
PR4					
PR5					
PR6					

CASE 8 DIAGNOSES

ICD-9-CM

DX1 Tendon rupture	8	4	4	.	8	
DX2				.		
DX3				.		
DX4				.		

CASE 8 PROCEDURES

CPT/HCPCS

PR1 Repair extensor tendon, leg; primary, without graft, each tendon	2	7	6	6	4
PR2					
PR3					
PR4					
PR5					
PR6					

CASE 9 DIAGNOSES   **ICD-9-CM**

DX1 Nonunion, tibia	7	3	3	.	8	2
DX2				.		
DX3				.		
DX4				.		

CASE 9 PROCEDURES   **CPT/HCPCS**

PR1 Split-thickness autograft, trunk, arms, legs; first 100 sq cm or less	1	5	1	0	0
PR2 Surgical preparation	1	5	0	0	2
PR3					
PR4					
PR5					
PR6					

CASE 10 DIAGNOSES   ICD-9-CM

DX1 Multiple myeloma	2	0	3	.	0	0
DX2				.		
DX3				.		
DX4				.		

CASE 10 PROCEDURES   CPT/HCPCS

PR1 Insertion of tunneled centrally inserted central venous catheter, without port or pump; age 5 or older	3	6	5	5	8
PR2					
PR3					
PR4					
PR5					
PR6					

CASE 11 DIAGNOSES

ICD-9-CM

DX1 End-stage renal disease	5	8	5	.	6	
DX2				.		
DX3				.		
DX4				.		

CASE 11 PROCEDURES

CPT/HCPCS

PR1 Arteriovenous anastomosis, open; by upper arm cephalic vein transposition	3	6	8	1	8
PR2					
PR3					
PR4					
PR5					
PR6					

CASE 12 DIAGNOSES ICD-9-CM

DX1 Congenital cataract	7	4	3	.	3	0
DX2				.		
DX3				.		
DX4				.		

CASE 12 PROCEDURES CPT/HCPCS

PR1 Extracapsular cataract removal with insertion of intraocular lens prothesis	6	6	9	8	2
PR2					
PR3					
PR4					
PR5					
PR6					

CASE 13 DIAGNOSES
ICD-9-CM

DX1 Diabetes mellitus	2	5	0	.	0	1
DX2 Delayed gastric emptying	5	3	6	.	8	
DX3 GI reflux	5	3	0	.	8	1
DX4				.		

CASE 13 PROCEDURES
CPT/HCPCS

PR1 Esophagus, gastroesophageal reflux test, nasal catheter pH electrode	9	1	0	3	4
PR2					
PR3					
PR4					
PR5					
PR6					

CASE 14 DIAGNOSES   **ICD-9-CM**

DX1 Status epilepticus	3	4	5	.	3	
DX2 Metastatic lung cancer	1	6	2	.	9	
DX3 Primary cancer, unknown	1	9	9	.	1	
DX4				.		

CASE 14 PROCEDURES   **CPT/HCPCS**

PR1 Electroencephalogram, awake and drowsy	9	5	8	1	6
PR2					
PR3					
PR4					
PR5					
PR6					

CASE 15 DIAGNOSES

ICD-9-CM

DX1 Klippel-Feil anomaly	7	5	6	.	1	6
DX2 Sprengel deformity	7	5	5	.	5	2
DX3 Ventricular septal defect	7	4	5	.	4	
DX4 Speech and language disorders	3	1	5	.	3	9

CASE 15 PROCEDURES

CPT/HCPCS

PR1 Auditory evoked potentials	9	2	5	8	5
PR2 Evoked otoacoustic emissions	9	2	5	8	7
PR3					
PR4					
PR5					
PR6					

CASE 16 DIAGNOSES   **ICD-9-CM**

DX1 Nerve palsy	3	7	8	.	5	3
DX2				.		
DX3				.		
DX4				.		

CASE 16 PROCEDURES   **CPT/HCPCS**

PR1 MRI, brain, with and without contrast	7	0	5	5	3
PR2					
PR3					
PR4					
PR5					
PR6					

Practice Exam 2 Answers

1. B   Retrovir is an antiretroviral which is used to treat viral infections including HIV infection which causes AIDS. For more information on Retrovir, see http://www.drugs.com/cdi/retrovir.html.

2. D   (Schraffenberger, 172.)

3. A   Histology refers to the tissue type of a lesion. The histology of tissue is determined by a pathologist and documented in the pathology report.

4. B   Patient may have several chronic conditions that co-exist at the time of their hospital admission and qualify as additional diagnoses. If there is documentation in the record to indicate the patient has a chronic condition, it should be coded. Chronic diseases treated on an ongoing basis may be coded and reported as many times as the patient receives treatment and care for the condition(s) (*ICD-9-CM Official Guidelines for Coding and Reporting, Section IV. Diagnostic Coding and Reporting Guidelines for Outpatient Services*).

5. C   The *ICD-9-CM Official Guidelines for Coding and Reporting, Section IV. Diagnostic Coding and Reporting Guidelines for Outpatient Services* indicate that when a physician qualifies a diagnostic statement as "probable," the condition qualified with that statement should not be coded as if it existed. Rather, the condition should be coded to the highest level of certainty such as the signs and symptoms the patient exhibits. The history of cholecystectomy has no relevance to the current encounter and should not be coded (Kuehn, 29–31).

6. D   Abnormal findings from laboratory results are not coded and reported unless the physician indicates their clinical significance. If the findings are outside the normal range and the physician has ordered other tests to evaluate the condition or has prescribed treatment, it is appropriate to ask the physician whether the diagnosis code(s) for the abnormal findings should be added (Schraffenberger, 256).

7. C   Progress notes are chronological statements about the patient's response to treatment during his or her stay at the facility (Kuehn, 10).

8. B   Vital signs are recorded as part of a physical examination (LaTour and Eichenwald Maki, 177).

9. A   Square brackets are used only in the Tabular List to enclose synonyms, alternative wordings, abbreviations, and explanatory phrases (Hazelwood and Venable, 25).

10. D   The use of a brace simplifies tabular entries and saves printing space by reducing repetitive working. A brace also connects a series of terms on the left or right with a statement on the other side of the brace (Hazelwood and Venable, 26).

11. B   For categories V30–V39 when a fourth digit "0—born in hospital" is used, there is a note that a fifth digit is required. These fifth digits refer to whether or not the baby was born via Cesarean section or not (Hazelwood and Venable, 38–39).

12. C   Epstein-Barr is a commonly known viral infection. The other choices listed are bacterial infections (Hazelwood and Venable, 74).

13. B   Code assignment for HIV depends on whether the patient is symptomatic or asymptomatic. Code 042, Human immunodeficiency virus [HIV] disease: Patients with HIV-related illness should be coded to 042. Category 042 includes AIDS, AIDS-like syndrome, AIDS-related complex, and symptomatic HIV infection (Hazelwood and Venable, 81).

14. A   ICD-9-CM defines "late effect" as the temporary or permanent condition that follows the acute phase of an illness or injury. In this case, "scarring following a burn"—the scar is the permanent condition following the injury (burn) (Hazelwood and Venable, 54).

15. D   ICD-9-CM provides the following coding guideline for burns: Classify burns of the same local site, but of different degrees, to the subcategory identifying the highest degree recorded in the diagnosis (Hazelwood and Venable, 252).

16. C   Category 948 is based on the classic "rule of nines" in estimating body surface involved: head and neck—9%; each arm—9%; each leg—18%; anterior trunk—18%; posterior trunk—18%, and genitalia—1% (Hazelwood and Venable, 253).

17. B   ICD-9-CM refers to medications (prescription or nonprescription) taken in combination with alcoholic beverages as a "poisoning" as opposed to an adverse effect (Hazelwood and Venable, 265).

18. D   In ICD-9-CM, mechanical complications include the mechanical breakdown/ displacement, leakage, mechanical obstruction, perforation, or protrusion of the device, implant, or graft (Hazelwood and Venable, 279).

19. A   In ICD-9-CM, hypersensitivities or allergic reactions that occur as qualitatively different responses to a drug, which are acquired only after re-exposure to the drug is the definition of an adverse effect (Hazelwood and Venable, 262).

20. D   A greenstick fracture is classified as a closed fracture. The sites of the fracture are the shafts of the tibia and fibula (Hazelwood and Venable, 247).

21. B   There are two sites to be coded—abdomen and right arm—both second-degree burn since this was the highest level of burn for each site. The fifth digit subclassification identifies the specific site (Hazelwood and Venable, 252–253).

22. B   Since the patient was postoperative, the postoperative infection code (998.59) should be coded as well as a code for the cellulitis of the leg which identifies the specific type of postoperative infection present (Hazelwood and Venable, 281–282).

23. B "Medicare covers colorectal barium enemas only in lieu of covered screening flexible sigmoidoscopies (HCPCS code G0104) or covered screening colonoscopies (HCPCS code G0105)" HHS, 130).

24. D When the coder compares the procedure description to the diagnosis description, there is a difference between the type of immunization being coded and the shoulder pain is linked to the cholesterol; therefore, the diagnosis was not correctly linked to the procedure (Kuehn, 305).

25. A Lacerations of the same site grouping and same complexity are added together for coding (Kuehn, 110).

26. C –LT and –RT are used to describe that x-rays are performed on each side (Kuehn, 209).

27. C Excisions of lesions are coded separately (Kuehn, 108–109).

28. D According to the Coding Guidelines, the service is a chemotherapy IV infusion of the initial substance, a sequential chemotherapy infusion, and a therapeutic injection (*CPT Professional Edition,* 486–490) (Kuehn, 253–255).

29. B Joint aspirations are an arthrocentesis (Kuehn, 121).

30. B The triangle ▲ is used to mark code descriptions that have changed (Kuehn, 16).

31. C The –76 modifier is used to indicate that a procedure is repeated by the same physician on the same day (Kuehn, 282).

32. A According to the Surgery Guidelines, the consultation to determine the need for the procedure is always excluded from the surgical global (*CPT Professional Edition,* 52) (Kuehn, 101–102).

33. C According to the Coding Guidelines, the –26 modifier is required because the pathologist is not employed by the facility and is billing separately. Each specimen must be reported separately (*CPT Professional Edition,* 422) (Kuehn, 228).

34. C The requirements for a consultation on a patient not covered by Medicare are met (Kuehn, 60–61).

35. B A removal of a portion of the patient's kidney is a partial nephrectomy (*CPT Assistant,* January 2003, 01:13, 9–21).

36. C This is an unstable finger fracture that requires manipulation but not percutaneous pinning (normally a day surgery procedure), or code 26725. In addition, the x-ray is of the fingers, not the hand, or code 73140.

37. A (Schraffenberger, 59–60.)

38. B The RBRVS system is the federal government's payment system for physicians. It is a system of classifying health services based on the cost of furnishing physicians' services in different settings, the skill and training levels required to perform the services, and the time and risk involved (Casto and Layman, 157).

39. A The revenue production report shows the number of times a particular procedure is coded and the total revenue produced as a result of the coding; it also identifies the most frequently used codes in the practice (Kuehn, 333–334).

40. B   A service distribution report can yield information about CPT/HCPCS coding patterns. It also provides data to identify problem areas in procedure coding (Kuehn, 328–329).

41. A   This is the definition of clustering. This practice could be considered fraudulent (Kuehn, 335).

42. B   The goal in claims submittal is to submit each claim as a clean claim which means it contains all of the required and accurate information. A clean claim is essential in order to receive timely and accurate reimbursement (Kuehn, 308).

43. C   For Medicare, a nonparticipating physician who does not accept assignment may not bill the patient more than the Medicare limiting charge, which is 115% of the Medicare approved amount (Kuehn, 297).

44. D   National coverage determinations (NCDs) or local coverage determinations (LCDs) are guidelines which specify what conditions or diagnoses are needed to justify specific services identified by CPT codes (Kuehn, 301–303).

45. C   In the hospital charges displayed, 8/13/20XX and 8/14/20XX are incorrectly coded with initial hospital service codes. The patient was seen in consultation on 8/12/20XX and took over the patient's care for the remainder of the admission, 8/13/20XX and 8/14/20XX should have been coded using subsequent hospital service codes (Kuehn, 58).

46. B   Only one initial hospital service code can be charged by the same physician during an inpatient stay.

47. B   Appendix B of the CPT book indicates additions, deletions, and revisions to codes for the current year. This is the best source of information to use in updating encounter forms (*CPT Professional Edition*, 534–543).

48. D   The CPT codes assigned for the cases scheduled as cervical discectomies are all from the lumbar section; therefore, coders would find a review of spinal anatomy helpful in their code assignments.

49. D   According to the E/M Service Guidelines, both the time spent counseling or coordinating care and the total time of the visit must be documented (*CPT Professional Edition*, 7) (Kuehn, 52).

50. B   The coder chose the correct medication but chose the wrong dosage. Depo-Provera is used for both contraception (at 150 mg) and for estrogen replacement therapy (at lower doses). Additional information on medroxyprogesterone acetate can be found at http://www.drugs.com/ppa/medroxyprogesterone-acetate.html.

51. C   Statements A, B, and D are actually disadvantages of using e-mail in the healthcare setting. However, using e-mail to clarify treatment instructions and medication administration is beneficial to patients and healthcare providers.

52. B   A database is a structure that allows for the storage of data about multiple entities (in this example, patients) and the relationship among the entities (LaTour and Eichenwald Maki, 125).

53. B   An encoder is a computer software program designed to assist coders in assigning appropriate clinical codes. An encoder helps ensure accurate reporting of diagnoses and procedures (LaTour and Eichenwald Maki, 400).

54. C   Electronic spreadsheets can be used to facilitate data collection and analysis. The advantage of spreadsheets is that charts and graphs can be formulated as the data are being analyzed.

55. C   Reliability refers to the consistency of any data set (LaTour and Eichenwald Maki, 343).

56. B   An amendment to the Federal False Claims Act offered financial incentives to informants, or "relators," who report providers to the government who are committing fraud. This reporting is known as a qui tam action (Hazelwood and Venable, 298).

57. B   Since the physician requesting the record is not listed as the surgeon on this case (or as the attending physician), the physician must have an authorization signed by the patient in order to review this record. This scenario is based on confidentiality and the patient's right (or invasion) of privacy (LaTour and Eichenwald Maki, 246).

58. B   The hospital does have a right to deny access if such access could possibly endanger the life or safety of a patient or another individual (Roach, 161).

59. C   The HIPAA Privacy Rule recognizes and incorporates the principle of "minimum necessary." Generally, only the minimum necessary amount of information necessary to fulfill the purpose of the request should be shared with internal users and external requestors (Abdelhak, 517).

60. D   The HIPAA Privacy Rule does not provide access to the patient for the following: oral information, psychotherapy notes, and information compiled in anticipation of, or for use in, a civil, criminal, or administrative action or proceeding (LaTour and Eichenwald Maki, 253).

CASE 1 DIAGNOSES

ICD-9-CM

DX1 Laceration of finger	8	8	3	.	0	
DX2				.		
DX3				.		
DX4				.		

CASE 1 PROCEDURES

CPT/HCPCS

PR1 Office and outpatient E/M, established	9	9	2	1	3
PR2 Wound repair, finger, 1.0 cm	1	2	0	0	1
PR3					
PR4					
PR5					
PR6					

CASE 2 DIAGNOSES   **ICD-9-CM**

DX1 Hematochezia	5	7	8	.	1	
DX2 Chronic renal insufficiency	5	8	5	.	9	
DX3 Interstitial pneumonitis	5	1	6	.	8	
DX4 Steroid-induced diabetes mellitus	2	5	1	.	8	

CASE 2 PROCEDURES   **CPT/HCPCS**

PR1 Inpatient consultation	9	9	2	5	5
PR2					
PR3					
PR4					
PR5					
PR6					

CASE 3 DIAGNOSES

ICD-9-CM

DX1 Epistaxis	7	8	4	.	7	
DX2				.		
DX3				.		
DX4				.		

CASE 3 PROCEDURES

CPT/HCPCS

PR1 Emergency department E/M	9	9	2	8	2
PR2 Control nasal hemorrhage, anterior, simple	3	0	9	0	1
PR3					
PR4					
PR5					
PR6					

CASE 4 DIAGNOSES ICD-9-CM

DX1 Septicemia	0	3	8	.	3	
DX2 Urinary tract infection	5	9	9	.	0	
DX3 Infection with *Providencia Stuartii*	0	4	1	.	8	4
DX4				.		

CASE 4 PROCEDURES CPT/HCPCS

PR1 Inpatient consultation	9	9	2	5	3
PR2					
PR3					
PR4					
PR5					
PR6					

CASE 5 DIAGNOSES   **ICD-9-CM**

DX1 Rib fractures	8	0	7	.	0	5
DX2 Pulmonary contusion	8	6	1	.	2	1
DX3 Hemopneumothorax	8	6	0	.	4	
DX4 Pubic rami fracture	8	0	8	.	2	

CASE 5 PROCEDURES   **CPT/HCPCS**

PR1 Initial hospital E/M	9	9	2	2	3
PR2					
PR3					
PR4					
PR5					
PR6					

CASE 6 DIAGNOSES   ICD-9-CM

DX1 Urinary tract infection	5	9	9	.	0	
DX2 Schizophrenia	2	9	5	.	9	0
DX3				.		
DX4				.		

CASE 6 PROCEDURES   CPT/HCPCS

PR1 Office and outpatient E/M, new	9	9	2	0	2
PR2 Pregnancy test	8	1	0	2	5
PR3 Urinalysis, automated with microscopy	8	1	0	0	1
PR4					
PR5					
PR6					

CASE 7 DIAGNOSES ICD-9-CM

DX1 Osteoarthritis of knee	7	1	5	.	9	6
DX2 Genu varum	7	3	6	.	4	2
DX3				.		
DX4				.		

CASE 7 PROCEDURES CPT/HCPCS

PR1 Arthroplasty, knee, condyle and plateau; Medial and lateral compartments	2	7	4	4	7
PR2 Computer-assisted musculoskeletal surgical navigational orthopedic procedure, imageless	2	0	9	8	5
PR3					
PR4					
PR5					
PR6					

CASE 8 DIAGNOSES   ICD-9-CM

DX1 Renal calculi	5	9	2	.	0	
DX2				.		
DX3				.		
DX4				.		

CASE 8 PROCEDURES   CPT/HCPCS

PR1 Percutaneous nephrostolithotomy or pyelostolithotomy	5	0	0	8	0
PR2					
PR3					
PR4					
PR5					
PR6					

CASE 9 DIAGNOSES   ICD-9-CM

DX1 Conn's syndrome	2	5	5	.	1	2
DX2 Hypertension	4	0	1	.	9	
DX3 Hypokalemia	2	7	6	.	8	
DX4				.		

CASE 9 PROCEDURES   CPT/HCPCS

PR1 Laparoscopy, surgical, with adrenalectomy, partial or complete	6	0	6	5	0
PR2					
PR3					
PR4					
PR5					
PR6					

CASE 10 DIAGNOSES   **ICD-9-CM**

DX1 Carcinoma in situ of breast	2	3	3	.	0	
DX2				.		
DX3				.		
DX4				.		

CASE 10 PROCEDURES   **CPT/HCPCS**

PR1 Mastectomy, partial; with axillary lymphadenectomy	1	9	3	0	2
PR2					
PR3					
PR4					
PR5					
PR6					

CASE 11 DIAGNOSES   **ICD-9-CM**

DX1 Congenital hypertrophic pyloric stenosis	7	5	0	.	5	
DX2 Thrombosed accessory spleen	7	5	9	.	0	
DX3				.		
DX4				.		

CASE 11 PROCEDURES   **CPT/HCPCS**

PR1 Laparoscopy, surgical, splenectomy	3	8	1	2	0
PR2 Unlisted laparoscopic procedure, stomach	4	3	6	5	9
PR3					
PR4					
PR5					
PR6					

CASE 12 DIAGNOSES   ICD-9-CM

DX1 Skin tag	7	0	1	.	9	
DX2 Preauricular sinus	7	4	4	.	4	6
DX3				.		
DX4				.		

CASE 12 PROCEDURES   CPT/HCPCS

PR1 Excision, benign lesion, excised diameter 1.1 cm to 2 cm	1	1	4	4	2
PR2 Removal of skin tags	1	1	2	0	0
PR3 Repair, intermediate wound, of face, ears, eyelids, nose, lips, and/or mucous membranes, 2.5 cm or less	1	2	0	5	1
PR4					
PR5					
PR6					

CASE 13 DIAGNOSES   ICD-9-CM

DX1 Intraocular foreign body	8	7	1	.	6	
DX2				.		
DX3				.		
DX4				.		

CASE 13 PROCEDURES   CPT/HCPCS

PR1 Removal of foreign body, intraocular; from posterior segment, nonmagnetic extraction	6	5	2	6	5
PR2 Removal of lens material; pars plana approach, with or without vitrectomy	6	6	8	5	2
PR3 Fitting of contact lens for treatment of disease	9	2	0	7	0
PR4 Monitoring of intraocular pressure during vitrectomy surgery	0	1	7	3	T
PR5					
PR6					

CASE 14 DIAGNOSES   **ICD-9-CM**

DX1 Acute bronchitis	4	6	6	.	0	
DX2 Hypertension	4	0	1	.	9	
DX3 Rheumatoid arthritis	7	1	4	.	0	
DX4 Type II diabetes mellitus	2	5	0	.	0	0

CASE 14 PROCEDURES   **CPT/HCPCS**

PR1 Office and outpatient E/M, new	9	9	2	0	3
PR2 Nebulizer treatment	9	4	6	4	0
PR3 Metered dose inhaler teaching	9	4	6	6	4
PR4 Albuterol and ipratropium bromide med	J	7	6	2	0
PR5					
PR6					

CASE 15 DIAGNOSES   **ICD-9-CM**

DX1 Palpitations	7	8	5	.	1	
DX2 History of surgery to heart and great vessels	V	1	5	.	1	
DX3				.		
DX4				.		

CASE 15 PROCEDURES   **CPT/HCPCS**

PR1 Electrocardiographic monitoring for 24 hrs, total service	9	3	2	2	4
PR2					
PR3					
PR4					
PR5					
PR6					

CASE 16 DIAGNOSES   **ICD-9-CM**

DX1 Hyperemesis gravidarum with electrolyte imbalance	6	4	3	.	1	3
DX2				.		
DX3				.		
DX4				.		

CASE 16 PROCEDURES   **CPT/HCPCS**

PR1 Basic metabolic panel	8	0	0	4	8
PR2 CBC with automated differential	8	5	0	2	5
PR3 Venipuncture	3	6	4	1	5
PR4					
PR5					
PR6					

Practice Exam 3 Answers

1. C   The PDR is the authoritative source of FDA-approved information on prescription drugs. It includes information on more than 3,000 brand name and generic drugs as well as information on usage, warning, and drug interactions.

2. A   (LaTour and Eichenwald Maki, 200.)

3. C   Physicians' orders drive the healthcare team. Orders may be for treatments, ancillary medical services, laboratory tests, radiological procedures, drugs, devices, restraints, or seclusion (LaTour and Eichenwald Maki, 196).

4. B   The location of the donor site is not needed to code grafts as the harvesting of the graft is included in the graft code. However, if the donor site requires skin grafting or local flaps, an additional code would be reported (Kuehn, 111–112).

5. C   (Kuehn, 62.)

6. B   The official *ICD-9-CM Coding Guidelines* are published quarterly in *Coding Clinic,* which is published by the Central Office on ICD-9-CM Coding of the American Hospital Association.

7. D   An eponym is defined as the naming of a disease, structure, operation, or procedure after the name of the person who discovered or first described it (Hazelwood and Venable, 15).

8. A   In the Tabular List, a colon is used after an incomplete term that needs one or more of the modifiers that follows so that it can be assigned to a given category or code (Hazelwood and Venable, 26).

9. C   All three volumes of ICD-9-CM use parentheses to enclose supplementary words or explanatory information that may or may not be present in the statement of a diagnosis or procedure (Hazelwood and Venable, 24).

10. B   In ICD-9-CM, a symptom is defined as any subjective evidence of disease reported by the patient to the physician (Hazelwood and Venable, 60).

11. D   The Official Guidelines state that the code for the underlying cause (infection or trauma) must be sequenced first (Hazelwood and Venable, 77).

12. A This occasion of service was only for the radiation therapy; therefore, it is sequenced before the code for the neoplasm (Hazelwood and Venable, 91).

13. C The diagnosis of hypercholesterolemia is to be sequenced first, followed by the obesity (Hazelwood and Venable, 104).

14. B The paranoid alcoholic psychosis is code followed by the alcohol dependence. The fifth digit "1" is for continuous use (Hazelwood and Venable, 120–121).

15. A The acute condition is sequenced first followed by the chronic condition (Hazelwood and Venable, 131–132).

16. B The primary diagnosis is the pernicious anemia with the agammaglobulinemia and gastritis being associated with the anemia and therefore placed after the anemia code (Hazelwood and Venable, 136).

17. A Code 404.01 addresses the hypertensive condition—stage III; 585.3 covers the kidney disease, stage III, and the remaining codes cover the diabetes and polyneuropathy (Hazelwood and Venable, 2010, 148).

18. D Maxillary sinusitis is coded to 461.0 and frontal sinusitis is coded to acute frontal sinusitis, 461.1 (Hazelwood and Venable, 169).

19. B This code is used because there was no mention of hemorrhage or perforation and was also without obstruction (Hazelwood and Venable, 181).

20. A In this case, both the code for the cystitis and the organism (E. coli) code must be used (Hazelwood and Venable, 192).

21. C (*CPT Professional Edition,* 59–60) (Kuehn, 109).

22. D The patient receives 600 mg of Rocephin. The HCPCS code description for J0696 is 250 mg. Therefore, 3 units of Rocephin must be reported (250 mg + 250 mg + some of the 3rd unit of 250 mg) (Kuehn, 254, 273).

23. A *Healthcare Common Procedural Coding System (HCPCS)* book or Physician Fee Schedule Relative Value File (CMS, 2010). This file contains all of the HCPCS codes and CPT codes, along with their relative values.

24. C The skin graft is coded as 15340 and the supply is coded as Q4101 × 15 units. Fifteen units are reported because the wound is 15 sq cm (5 × 3) (Kuehn, 111–113).

25. D Replacement casts are coded separately (*CPT Professional Edition,* 139) (Kuehn, 126).

26. A The codes required for this case are the left heart catheterization, the injection procedure, and the imaging procedure (Kuehn, 240–241).

27. A All of the work described is included in code 29881 (Kuehn, 127).

28. B The procedure described is a colonoscopy with biopsy and is coded as 45380 (Kuehn, 151).

29. D When the office only performs the x-ray (the technical component), and the physician reading the x-ray is from another group, the –TC modifier is applied to the x-ray code (Kuehn, 208–209).

30. A   Index entry under Repair, Anal fistula (*CPT Professional Edition,* 729).

31. C   The only correct answer of these four is C, stating that you code all the laceration repairs (by adding together the lengths of those of the same site and complexity) and listing the code for the most complex repair first (Kuehn, 110).

32. B   A cast application is included in the closed treatment of the trimalleolar ankle fracture (*CPT Professional Edition,* 139) (Kuehn, 126).

33. B   *CPT Assistant* is the official source for guidance on how to assign a CPT code.

34. C   (*Dorland's Medical Dictionary*—computerized tomography, 1919).

35. C   Refer to the chart in CPT to see that 115 minutes of critical care is coded using 3 codes (*CPT Professional Edition,* 22).

36. B   Modifiers would not be appended to unlisted codes because these codes describe new or unclassified procedures that have no standard description. Therefore, the description does not need to be modified (Kuehn, 278).

37. D   The government will pay 80%, or $104, of the Medicare PAR approved amount (AMA 2008, 79).

38. D   The government will pay 95% of the Medicare PAR payment of $80, or a total of $76. (95% of the 80% of the approved amount) (AMA 2008, 79).

39. C   The patient is responsible for 20%, or $19, of the Medicare approved amount (AMA 2008, 79).

40. B   (Work RVU × work GPCI) + (practice expense RVU × practice expense GPCI) + (malpractice RVU × malpractice GPCI) × $36.0666 = (1.00 × 1.0) + (0.5 × 1.5) + (0.02 × 1.0) = 1 + .75 + .02 = 1.77; 1.77 × 36.0666 = $63.84 (AMA, 70).

41. D   The physician will not receive any payment from the federal government; the patient is responsible for the entire bill (AMA 2008, 79).

42. B   A non-PAR who does not accept assignment is bound by the limiting charge rule of the government. The limiting charge is 115% of the non-PAR approved amount, which in this case is 115% of $166.25 (95% of $175) or $191.18 (AMA 2008, 79).

43. B   Practice expense is the overhead costs of the practice such as office rent, wages of nonphysician personnel, supplies, and equipment (Glass, 9).

44. D   The first step in claims appeal is called redetermination, which is a claims review by an individual who was not involved in the initial claim review determination. This request must be made within 120 days of receiving the initial claim determination (Valerius, et al., 465).

45. C   Unbundling is the practice of coding services separately that should be coded together as a package because all parts are included within one code and therefore, one price. Unbundling done deliberately could be considered fraud (Kuehn, 335).

46. C   The documentation states that the laceration was closed with one simple stitch. This does not support the assignment of the code for a complex repair that was listed on the encounter summary.

47. B   The –25 modifier should be assigned to the E/M code if a significant, separately identifiable E/M service is performed by the same physician on the same day as a procedure (Kuehn, 279).

48. C   The service distribution report is frequently used for this purpose (Kuehn, 328).

49. C   The immunization administration codes are missing (*CPT Professional Edition,* 435–436) (Kuehn, 240).

50. C   The charge summary is sometimes called the office service report and contains a summary of all billing data entered for the practice on one day (Kuehn, 324).

51. C   In this example, 10 splints are no longer available in stock. The coding manager can only assume that these splints were provided to patients and that physicians did not code them. Therefore, the appropriate action is to talk with the physicians about the use of supplies and the need for coding.

52. D   Electronic data interchange (EDI) is the electronic transfer of information such as health claims transmitted electronically in a standard format between trading partners. EDI allows entities within the healthcare system to exchange medical, billing, and other information and to process transactions in a manner that is fast and cost effective (LaTour and Eichenwald Maki, 180).

53. C   An intranet is a private information network that is similar to the Internet and who servers are located inside a firewall or security barrier so that the general public cannot gain access to information housed within the network (LaTour and Eichenwald Maki, 758).

54. B   Interoperability is the ability, generally by adoption of standards, of computer systems to work together.

55. B   HIPAA provides for criminal penalties for healthcare professional who "knowingly and willingly" attempt to defraud any health program 9 Hazelwood and Venable, 2010, 298).

56. C   The OIG investigates and prosecutes individuals who overbill Medicare and also develops an annual "work plan" that lists specific "target areas" monitored in a given year (Hazelwood and Venable, 299).

57. C   Receiving kickbacks in exchange for referring patients to specific facilities is one of the examples listed under the definition of fraud (Hazelwood and Venable, 299).

58. A   *Federal Register,* 58400 (63:210. Oct. 30, 1998). Providers who voluntarily report fraudulent conduct need to use the Provider Self-Disclosure Protocol form.

59. D   Validity refers to the accuracy of the data (LaTour and Eichenwald Maki, 342–343).

60. B   The Stark Law prohibits a physician from referring patients to an entity for services paid for by federal or state health benefits programs if a physician has a financial relationship with the entity (Roach, 481).

CASE 1 DIAGNOSES | ICD-9-CM

DX1 Spinal stenosis, thoracic region	7	2	4	.	0	1
DX2 Trochanteric bursitis	7	2	6	.	5	
DX3 Trigger finger	7	2	7	.	0	3
DX4				.		

CASE 1 PROCEDURES | CPT/HCPCS

PR1 Office and outpatient E/M, established	9	9	2	1	4
PR2 Injection, small joint	2	0	6	0	0
PR3 Triamcinolone medication, 10 mg	J	3	3	0	1
PR4 Injection, major joint	2	0	6	1	0
PR5 Injection, major joint	2	0	6	1	0
PR6					

CASE 2 DIAGNOSES   **ICD-9-CM**

DX1 Transient ischemic attack	4	3	5	.	9	
DX2 Mitral valve prolapse	4	2	4	.	0	
DX3				.		
DX4				.		

CASE 2 PROCEDURES   **CPT/HCPCS**

PR1 Emergency department E/M	9	9	2	8	5
PR2 EKG interpretation	9	3	0	1	0
PR3					
PR4					
PR5					
PR6					

CASE 3 DIAGNOSES   **ICD-9-CM**

DX1 Biliary colic	5	7	4	.	2	0
DX2				.		
DX3				.		
DX4				.		

CASE 3 PROCEDURES   **CPT/HCPCS**

PR1 Outpatient consultation	9	9	2	4	4
PR2					
PR3					
PR4					
PR5					
PR6					

CASE 4 DIAGNOSES   **ICD-9-CM**

DX1 Multiple rib fractures	8	0	7	.	0	9
DX2 Hemothorax	8	6	0	.	2	
DX3 Ulnar fracture	8	1	3	.	0	4
DX4 Abrasions, chest wall	9	1	1	.	0	

CASE 4 PROCEDURES   **CPT/HCPCS**

PR1 Initial hospital E/M	9	9	2	2	3
PR2					
PR3					
PR4					
PR5					
PR6					

CASE 5 DIAGNOSES   **ICD-9-CM**

DX1 COPD/chronic bronchitis	4	9	1	.	2	1
DX2 Lymphocytic leukemia	2	0	4	.	1	0
DX3				.		
DX4				.		

CASE 5 PROCEDURES   **CPT/HCPCS**

PR1 Office and outpatient E/M, established	9	9	2	1	4
PR2					
PR3					
PR4					
PR5					
PR6					

CASE 6 DIAGNOSES   **ICD-9-CM**

DX1 Fracture aftercare	V	5	4	.	1	1
DX2 Still's syndrome	7	1	4	.	3	0
DX3				.		
DX4				.		

CASE 6 PROCEDURES   **CPT/HCPCS**

PR1 Office and outpatient E/M, new	9	9	2	0	1
PR2 Hardware removal, superficial	2	0	6	7	0
PR3					
PR4					
PR5					
PR6					

CASE 7 DIAGNOSES   **ICD-9-CM**

DX1 Carotid stenosis	4	3	3	. 1	0
DX2				.	
DX3				.	
DX4				.	

CASE 7 PROCEDURES   **CPT/HCPCS**

PR1 Thromboendarterectomy with or without patch graft; carotid, vertebral, subclavian, by neck incision	3	5	3	0	1
PR2					
PR3					
PR4					
PR5					
PR6					

CASE 8 DIAGNOSES

ICD-9-CM

DX1 Mucocele (lesion), lower lip	5	2	8	▪	5	
DX2				▪		
DX3				▪		
DX4				▪		

CASE 8 PROCEDURES

CPT/HCPCS

PR1 Excision of lesion of mucosa and submucosa, vestibule of mouth, with simple repair	4	0	8	1	2
PR2					
PR3					
PR4					
PR5					
PR6					

CASE 9 DIAGNOSES   ICD-9-CM

DX1 Metastatic disease, femoral neck	1	9	8	.	5	
DX2 Renal cell carcinoma	1	8	9	.	0	
DX3 Pathologic fracture, femur	7	3	3	.	1	4
DX4				.		

CASE 9 PROCEDURES   CPT/HCPCS

PR1 Open treatment of femoral fracture	2	7	2	3	6
PR2 Prophylactic treatment of femur	2	7	4	9	5
PR3 Partial excision bone, femur	2	7	3	6	0
PR4					
PR5					
PR6					

CASE 10 DIAGNOSES | ICD-9-CM

DX1 Orbital pseudotumor	3	7	6	.	1	1
DX2				.		
DX3				.		
DX4				.		

CASE 10 PROCEDURES | CPT/HCPCS

PR1 Biopsy of lacrimal gland	6	8	5	1	0
PR2					
PR3					
PR4					
PR5					
PR6					

CASE 11 DIAGNOSES

ICD-9-CM

DX1 Middle ear cholesteatoma	3	8	5	.	3	2
DX2				.		
DX3				.		
DX4				.		

CASE 11 PROCEDURES

CPT/HCPCS

PR1 Tympanoplasty with mastoidectomy	6	9	6	4	3
PR2					
PR3					
PR4					
PR5					
PR6					

CASE 12 DIAGNOSES

ICD-9-CM

DX1 Rejection of kidney transplant	9	9	6	.	8	1
DX2 End-stage renal disease	5	8	5	.	6	
DX3				.		
DX4				.		

CASE 12 PROCEDURES

CPT/HCPCS

PR1 Removal of transplanted renal allograft	5	0	3	7	0
PR2					
PR3					
PR4					
PR5					
PR6					

CASE 13 DIAGNOSES   **ICD-9-CM**

DX1 Other current conditions classifiable elsewhere	6	4	8	.	9	3
DX2 Carpal tunnel syndrome	3	5	4	.	0	
DX3				.		
DX4				.		

CASE 13 PROCEDURES   **CPT/HCPCS**

PR1 Needle electromyography; one extremity	9	5	8	6	0
PR2 Nerve conduction, amplitude and latency/velocity study, each nerve, motor (median)	9	5	9	0	0
PR3 Nerve conduction, amplitude and latency/velocity study, each nerve, motor (ulnar)	9	5	9	0	0
PR4 Nerve conduction, amplitude and latency/velocity study, each nerve, sensory (median)	9	5	9	0	4
PR5 Nerve conduction, amplitude and latency/velocity study, each nerve, sensory (ulnar)	9	5	9	0	4
PR6					

CASE 14 DIAGNOSES

ICD-9-CM

DX1 Cellulitis, leg	6	8	2	.	6	
DX2 Diabetes	2	5	0	.	7	0
DX3 Peripheral vascular disease	4	4	3	.	8	1
DX4				.		

CASE 14 PROCEDURES

CPT/HCPCS

PR1 Office and outpatient E/M, established	9	9	2	1	3
PR2 IV push	9	6	3	7	4
PR3 Rocephin 250 mg	J	0	6	9	6
PR4 Rocephin 250 mg	J	0	6	9	6
PR5 Rocephin 250 mg	J	0	6	9	6
PR6 Rocephin 250 mg	J	0	6	9	6

CASE 15 DIAGNOSES   ICD-9-CM

DX1 Chemotherapy treatment	V	5	8	.	1	1
DX2 Ovarian cancer	1	8	3	.	0	
DX3 Metastatic lung cancer	1	9	7	.	0	
DX4				.		

CASE 15 PROCEDURES   CPT/HCPCS

PR1 Chemotherapy infusion, 1st hour	9	6	4	1	3
PR2 Carboplatin 50 mg	J	9	0	4	5
PR3 Chemotherapy infusion, additional hour	9	6	4	1	7
PR4 Paclitaxel 30 mg	J	9	2	6	5
PR5 IV infusion, 1st hour	9	6	3	6	7
PR6 Ondansetron 1 mg	J	2	4	0	5

CASE 16 DIAGNOSES ICD-9-CM

DX1 Dental Caries	5	2	1	.	0	3
DX2 Status post, liver transplant	V	4	2	.	7	
DX3				.		
DX4				.		

CASE 16 PROCEDURES CPT/HCPCS

PR1 Extraction, tooth K	D	7	1	4	0
PR2 Extraction, tooth S	D	7	1	4	0
PR3 Extraction, tooth T	D	7	1	4	0
PR4					
PR5					
PR6					

References

The following resources are referenced in the answer key:

Abdelhak, M. 2007. *Health Information: Management of a Strategic Resource*. St. Louis, MO: Saunders Elsevier.

American Health Information Management Association. 2010. *Pocket Glossary for Health Information Management and Technology*, 2nd ed. Chicago: AHIMA.

American Health Information Management Association House of Delegates. 2008 (September). AHIMA Standards of Ethical Coding. Chicago: AHIMA.

American Medical Association. 2010. *CPT Professional Edition*, 2010: Chicago: AMA.

American Medical Association. 2010. *CPT Changes 2010: An Insider's View*. Chicago: AMA.

American Medical Association. 2008. *Medicare RBRVS: The Physicians' Guide*. Chicago: AMA.

American Medical Association. *CPT Assistant*, 1990 through 2010 editions. Chicago: AMA.

Brodnik, M. 2009. *Fundamentals of Law for Health Informatics and Information Management*. Chicago: AHIMA.

Brown, F. 2010. *ICD-9-CM Coding Handbook with Answers*. Chicago: American Hospital Association.

Casto, A. and E. Layman. 2006. *Principles of Healthcare Reimbursement*. Chicago: AHIMA.

Centers for Medicare and Medicaid Services, Department of Health and Human Services. 2010. Physician Fee Schedule Relative Value. http://www.cms.hhs.gov/PhysicianFeeSched/PFSRVF/list.asp#TopOfPage.

Centers for Medicare and Medicaid Services and the National Center for Health Statistics. 2008. *ICD-9-CM Official Guidelines for Coding and Reporting*. http://www.cdc.gov/nchs/datawh/ftpserv/ftpICD9/icdguide08.pdf.

Department of Health and Human Services (HHS). 2007 (August). *The Guide to Medicare Preventive Services for Physicians, Providers, Suppliers and Other Healthcare Professionals*, 2nd ed., August, 2007, 130. http://www.cms.hhs.gov/MLNProducts/downloads/mps_guide_web-061305.pdf.

Dorland's Illustrated Medical Dictionary, 30th ed. 2003. St. Louis, MO: Saunders Elsevier.

Glass, K. 2008. *RVUs: Applications for Medical Practice Success*, 2nd ed. Englewood, CO: Medical Group Management Association.

Hazelwood, A. and C. Venable. 2010. *ICD-9-CM Diagnostic Coding and Reimbursement for Physician Services*. Chicago: AHIMA.

Ingenix. 2010. *Coder's Desk Reference for Procedures 2010*. Salt Lake City, UT: Ingenix.

Kuehn, L. 2010. *Procedural Coding and Reimbursement for Physician Services: Applying Current Procedural Terminology and HCPCS*. Chicago: AHIMA.

LaTour, K.M. and S. Eichenwald Maki, eds. 2010. *Health Information Management Concepts, Principles, and Practice*, 3rd ed. Chicago: AHIMA.

Roach, W. et al. 2006. *Medical Records and the Law*. Sudbury, MA: Jones and Bartlett.

Schraffenberger, L. 2010. *Basic ICD-9-CM Coding*. Chicago: AHIMA.

Valerius, J. et al. 2008. *Medical Insurance: An Integrated Claims Process Approach*. Boston: McGraw-Hill.